Cardiovascular Disease Matters in Primary Care

Ruth Chambers

Gill Wakley

and

Zafar Iqbal

Forewords by

Richard Baker

and

Lynn Young

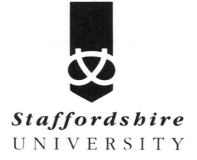

Staffordshire
UNIVERSITY

RADCLIFFE MEDICAL PRESS

Radcliffe Medical Press Ltd
18 Marcham Road, Abingdon, Oxon OX14 1AA

British Library Cataloguing in Publication Data

A catalogue record for this book is available from the British Library.

ISBN 1 85775 419 0

Typeset by Joshua Associates Ltd, Oxford
Printed and bound by TJ International Ltd, Padstow, Cornwall

Contents

Foreword

Clinical governance is a new idea, and it will take several years before we can claim to fully understand its methods and implications. But there should be no mistake – it is a big idea. By making health service organisations and their leaders accountable for the quality of care, a new way of thinking and behaving is beginning to emerge in the NHS. In time, and as the Commission for Health Improvement works through its programme of inspections, we are going to become more aware of how clinical governance will affect the operation of health services and professional practice.

Cardiovascular disease accounts for more mortality and morbidity than any other disease. And much of the responsibility for the prevention of cardiovascular disease rests with primary care, as does the lion's share of the long-term management of established illness. Inevitably, therefore, this book will be of great relevance to members of primary healthcare teams. The authors have not simply written a book for quiet evening reading, however. You should do more with it than read it. It contains direct, practical advice in relation to each of the key cardiovascular disorders, and guidance on developing your own personal development plan and the practice learning plan. It is therefore a book to 'do', or interact with, rather than just read. Make use of this book and you will start to release the full potential of clinical governance and will improve the care of people at risk of, or with, cardiovascular problems.

Professor Richard Baker
Director
Clinical Governance Research & Development Unit
Department of General Practice & Primary Health Care
University of Leicester
May 2001

Foreword

This book will prove to be of huge value to the many doctors, nurses and other disciplines who have a collective determination to improve the primary and secondary prevention and treatment of cardiovascular disease.

While hospital treatment continues to hold on to the main focus of attention from both the media and politicians there is also a consensus that high-quality primary healthcare services make a profound difference to cardiovascular morbidity and mortality.

Making a positive difference to cardiovascular disease means that all primary healthcare disciplines need to integrate their particular activities and, as a team, focus on doing 'the right thing at the right time in the right place'. It is only by mobilising all disciplines to concentrate their efforts, skills, talents and knowledge on doing the right thing that the full potential can be achieved. While the National Service Framework (NSF) for coronary heart disease provides the platform for ensuring that the right care is provided, people are hungry for more help.

The authors have worked hard to achieve the right help for the many people working in primary healthcare who are committed to making their contribution to winning the battle against cardiovascular disease.

Cardiovascular Disease Matters in Primary Care clarifies how the recommendations made in the NSF can be implemented and, as a result, can help people to believe that better, more effective care is possible. Most importantly, readers will also gain the essential confidence to know that they are, indeed, doing the right thing!

Primary care is going through a time of overwhelming change, transformation and development. For some clinicians a sense of hopelessness and exhaustion is a reality. To these people, in particular, this book is highly commended. Practical advice, information and useful case studies are available to the reader. Translating the content of the book to practice within general practice and community health services is possible. The book narrows the gap between theory and practice, and will encourage primary healthcare enthusiasts to believe that they have the potential to improve community health. Another knock-on effect will be a large number of newly motivated primary healthcare teams and a high level of job satisfaction! Many congratulations to the authors.

Lynn Young
Community Health Adviser
Royal College of Nursing
May 2001

About the authors

Ruth Chambers has been a GP for 20 years and is currently Professor of Primary Care Development at Staffordshire University. She has designed and organised many types of educational initiatives, including distance-learning programmes. Recently she has developed a keen interest in working with GPs, nurses and others in primary care around clinical governance and practice personal and professional development plans. Ruth is co-authoring this new series of books designed to help readers draw up their own personal development plans or practice learning plans around important clinical topics, such as cardiovascular disease.

Gill Wakley started in general practice in 1966, but transferred to community medicine shortly afterwards and then into public health. A desire for increased contact with patients caused a move back into general practice, together with community gynaecology, in 1978. She has been combining the two in varying amounts ever since. Throughout she has been heavily involved in learning and teaching. She was in a training general practice, became an instructing doctor and a regional assessor in family planning, and was until recently a senior clinical lecturer with the Primary Care Department at Keele University. Like Ruth, she has run all types of educational initiatives and activities, from individual mentoring and instruction, to small group work, plenary lectures, distance-learning programmes, work-shops, and courses for a wide range of health professionals and lay people.

Zafar Iqbal entered public health medicine after completing a general practice vocational training scheme in 1989. He became a public health consultant at South Staffordshire Health Authority in 1994, and is currently also an honorary senior lecturer in public health medicine at Birmingham University. In the last few years he has recommenced his career in general practice on a sessional basis. He is currently leading the implementation of the Coronary Heart Disease National Service Framework within South Staffordshire, and is a member of the West Midlands Regional Cardiac Forum. He has recently been involved in a variety of initiatives to promote a more systematic approach to the management of coronary heart disease in the primary care setting. His other main interest is clinical governance and how this links in with delivering the National Service Frameworks.

Acknowledgements

We should like to thank the Radcliffe Medical Press team for all the effort they have put into producing this new series of books, especially Jamie Etherington for editing and Gill Nineham for commissioning the series, and Gregory Moxon and Angela Jones for promoting the material. They have really supported us as authors, and have fast-tracked the publication of the books so that the contents are as up to date as possible.

Ruth Chambers
Gill Wakley
Zafar Iqbal

List of abbreviations

ACE	angiotensin-converting enzyme
AF	atrial fibrillation
BMI	body mass index
CABG	coronary artery bypass graft
CHD	coronary heart disease
COPD	chronic obstructive pulmonary disease
CPN	community psychiatric nurse
CVD	cardiovascular disease
DVT	deep venous thrombosis
HDL	high-density lipoprotein
Hg	mercury
HImP	health improvement programme
IT	information technology
LDL	low-density lipoprotein
MI	myocardial infarction
NHS	National Health Service
NNT	number needed to treat
NSF	National Service Framework
NYHA	New York Heart Association
PAM	professions allied to medicine
PCG	primary care group
PCO	primary care organisation
PCT	primary care trust
PDP	personal development plan
PPDP	practice personal and professional development plan
PTCA	percutaneous transluminal coronary angioplasty
SWOT	strengths, weaknesses, opportunities and threats
TIA	transient ischaemic attack

Introduction

This book sets out how learning more about cardiovascular disease and reviewing your current practice can be incorporated into your personal development plan or the practice learning plan.[1]

You need to develop a dual focus on improving the clinical management of cardiovascular disease (CVD) and improving the efficiency of your working environment. Practice team members should work together to direct their individual personal learning plans to form their practice personal and professional development plan. This should complement the clinical governance and business plans of the practice or primary care organisation.[2]

We are using the term 'primary care organisation' in this book to include primary care groups or trusts in England, local health groups in Wales, local health care co-operatives in Scotland and local health and social care groups in Northern Ireland.

Coronary heart disease (CHD) is the single commonest cause of death in the UK. It accounted for nearly a quarter of all deaths in the UK in 1996 – 28% of deaths in men and 18% of deaths in women. Each year about 300 000 people have heart attacks in the UK, and only half of them survive. About 1.4 million people suffer from heart disease, including angina, and a high proportion of these are relatively young people.

Facts about coronary heart disease

- The premature death rate from CHD for South Asians living in the UK is 46% higher than the average for men and 51% higher than the average for women.
- Coronary heart disease caused 150 000 deaths in the UK in 1996.
- The death rate from coronary heart disease in the UK is among the highest in the world. Only Ireland, Hungary and some eastern European countries have higher death rates.
- The decline in death rates from heart disease has been slower among women than among men. Coronary heart disease death rates fell by 22% in women, compared with 27% in men, in England between 1983 and 1993.

It is estimated that 4% of all consultations in general practice are at least partly related to prevention and/or treatment of coronary heart disease. The cost to general practice of these consultations (excluding prescribing costs) was estimated to be £57.9 million for the UK in 1996.

Stroke is important because it is the third commonest cause of death in the developed world. Although a stroke can occur at any age, half of all strokes occur in people over 70 years of age. About 10% of people with an ischaemic stroke die within the first month, and about 50% of the survivors still have some disability after the first 6 months.

The reasons for focusing on CHD are that not only is it the single commonest cause of death in the UK, but also much of the morbidity and premature mortality is preventable. About three million people have symptomatic coronary heart disease. Reducing the death rate from coronary heart disease, stroke and related diseases in people under 75 years of age by at least 40% would save up to 200000 lives in England alone – the target set by the English government to be reached by 2010.[3]

In England, the National Service Framework (NSF) for Coronary Heart Disease has set out milestones with goals and standards for the strategic development of coronary heart disease services.[4] These national standards will be delivered through clinical governance and local health improvement programmes. The Centre for Health Improvement (CHI), the NHS performance framework and the NHS patient survey will monitor the standards.

The NSF for Coronary Heart Disease aims to tackle the delays in service delivery at critical points in the care pathway such as the following:

- for patients with suspected heart attacks, delays in contacting emergency care and therefore accessing thrombolysis
- unacceptable delays between the time when the GP identifies CHD symptoms and the time when the patient receives specialist care
- delays between initial GP referral and the first out-patient appointment
- delays between clinical attendance and diagnosis
- delays between diagnosis and completion of investigations, with further delays in instituting appropriate treatment.

Integrated cardiac care is central to the redesign of the coronary heart disease services in line with the NSF for Coronary Heart Disease to provide initial accurate and prompt diagnoses, rapid-response emergency care, improved access to specialist services, personalised consistent care, and enhanced cardiac rehabilitation and palliative care. It concentrates on the following areas:

- secondary prevention, which includes health promotion activities such as smoking cessation services
- a streamlined system for the care of patients with suspected myocardial infarction
- the proper assessment and care of patients with angina
- the improved management of patients with heart failure
- improved cardiac revascularisation and rehabilitation.

You may decide to allocate 50% of the time you intend to spend drawing up and applying a personal development plan in any one year to learning more about cardiovascular disease. That would leave space in your learning plan for other important topics such as mental health, diabetes or cancer – whatever is a priority for you, your post and your patient population. There will be some overlap between topics – you cannot consider a patient with diabetes in isolation from their cardio-vascular risk factors, and that means understanding and knowing how to prevent and manage diabetes and cardiovascular problems, too.

The first chapter of the book describes how a clinical governance culture incorporates effective clinical management and well-organised working conditions. You should be able to demonstrate that you are fit to practise as an individual clinician or manager (best practice in the management of cardiovascular disease in this case), and that your working environment is fit to practise from. This section will be relevant to all readers, whether they are clinicians or primary care managers, so that they understand more of the context within which they work and how their individual contribution fits into the whole picture of healthcare.

Thereafter, each chapter gradually builds up your knowledge base of cardiovascular disease so that you know how to access the most recent evidence for hypertension, angina, myocardial infarction, stroke, atrial fibrillation and the secondary and primary prevention of cardiovascular disease.

The whole programme builds up to the construction of a personal development plan and a practice personal and professional develop-ment plan in Chapters 9 and 10.[1] Interactive reflection exercises at the end of each chapter give the reader an opportunity to assess their learning needs, review their performance or that of the practice organisation, and reflect on what improvements to make. You might want to complete a selection of the reflection exercises, or all of them. You might have other ideas for exercises to identify your own learning needs or gaps in the practice team performance. The main thing is to reflect on what you have learned and to apply that learning in practice.

You should transfer information from these needs assessment exercises to the relevant slots in your personal development plan, or to your practice personal and professional development plan if you are working as a team. Adopt a wide-based approach to improving quality – think of how you are establishing a clinical governance culture in your own practice team in your timed action plans.

What should you do next?

Study the template for a personal development plan on pages 142–151 or a practice personal and professional development plan on pages 165–172. You will be filling this in as you go along. Decide whether you will be starting out on your personal development plan or working with colleagues on the practice learning plan. Everyone's personal development plans should mesh with the practice learning plan by the time you have finished drawing them up.

Make changes as a result – to your workplace, or to the equipment in your practice, or to the advice you give patients, or to the way in which you manage and investigate coronary heart disease or complicating problems.

References

1 Wakley G, Chambers R and Field S (2000) *Continuing Professional Development: making it happen.* Radcliffe Medical Press, Oxford.
2 Chambers R and Wakley G (2000) *Making Clinical Governance Work for You.* Radcliffe Medical Press, Oxford.
3 Secretary of State for Health (1999) *Saving Lives: our healthier nation.* Department of Health, London.
4 NHS Executive (2000) *National Service Framework for Coronary Heart Disease.* Department of Health, London.

CHAPTER 1

Clinical governance and the management of cardiovascular disease

Clinical governance is about doing anything and everything required to maximise the quality of healthcare or services provided for, and received by, individual patients or the general population – in this case, those with cardiovascular disease or at risk from it.[1,2]

We should be able to use clinical governance to improve the detection and control of chronic conditions such as cardiovascular disease. Clinical governance is inclusive – making quality everyone's business, whether they are a doctor, a nurse or other health professional, a manager, a member of staff or a strategic planner. Good healthcare relies on the multidisciplinary team to support the person with cardiovascular disease in self-managing their disease in as much as they are able to do so. Delivering best practice requires sufficient clinical staff who are up to date and relate well to their patients, working with efficient systems and procedures that are patient friendly.

Components of clinical governance[2]

The components of clinical governance are not new. However, bringing them together under the banner of clinical governance and introducing more explicit accountability for performance is a new style of working.

The following 14 themes are core components of professional and service development which together form a comprehensive approach to providing high-quality healthcare services and clinical governance.[2] These are illustrated in Figure 1.1.

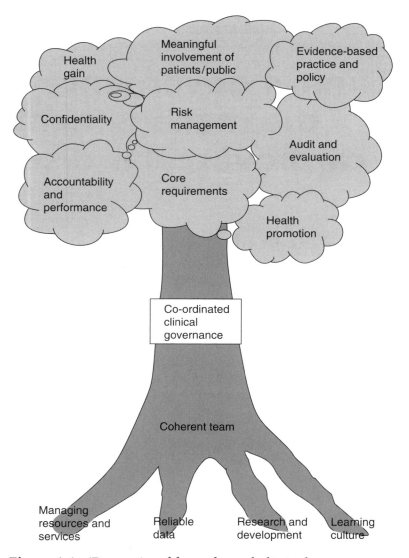

Figure 1.1: 'Routes' and branches of clinical governance.

If you interweave these 14 components into your individual and workplace-based personal and professional development plans you will have addressed the requirements for clinical governance at the same time.

1 *Learning culture*: for patients and staff in the practice or primary care organisation or in secondary care.
2 *Research and development culture*: in the practice or throughout the health service.

3 *Reliable and accurate data*: in the practice, across the primary care organisation and across the NHS as a seamless whole.

4 *Well-managed resources and services*: as individuals, as a practice, across the NHS and in conjunction with other organisations.

5 *Coherent team*: well-integrated teams within a practice, including attached staff.

6 *Meaningful involvement of patients and the public*: including those with cardiovascular disease, those who care for them and the general population.

7 *Health gain*: from improving the health of staff and patients in a practice, between practices and in a primary care organisation.

8 *Confidentiality*: of information at the reception desk, in consultations, in medical notes, between practitioners and with the outside world.

9 *Evidence-based practice and policy*: applying it in practice, in the district and across the NHS.

10 *Accountability and performance*: for standards, performance of individuals and the practice – both to the public and to those in authority.

11 *Core requirements*: good fit with skill mix, and whether individuals are competent to do their jobs, as well as communication, workforce numbers and morale at practice level.

12 *Health promotion*: for patients, the public, your staff and colleagues – opportunistic and in general, or targeting those with most needs.

13 *Audit and evaluation*: for instance, of the extent to which individuals and practice teams adhere to best practice in clinical management.

14 *Risk management*: being competent to spot those at risk, and reducing risks and probabilities of ill health. Risk management is really important at all stages of the clinical management of cardiovascular disease.

The challenges to delivering clinical governance

Delivering high-quality healthcare, with guaranteed minimum standards of care at all times, is a major challenge. At present the quality of healthcare is patchy and variable. We are not very good at detecting under-performance and rectifying it at an early stage. The small number of clinicians who do under-perform exert a disproportionately large effect on the public's confidence. Causes of under-performance in an individual might be a result of a lack of knowledge or skills, poor attitudes or ill health or a lack of resources. Poor management is nearly always a contributory reason for inadequate clinical services.

We need to understand why variation exists and explore ways of reducing inequalities. Variation in the quality of healthcare provided is common – between different practices in the same locality, between staff of the same discipline working in the same practice or unit, and between care given to some groups of the population rather than others.

Clinical governance offers a co-ordinated approach to overcoming these areas of risk.[3] The complex cultural change that will be required to deliver uniformly excellent care is immense. We need to develop measurable outcomes that professionals, patients and the public consider to be relevant and meaningful. Then we can assess the progress made through implementing clinical governance in the milestones and targets set out in the National Service Framework for Coronary Heart Disease.

Box 1.1

Coronary heart disease is well suited to act as a tracer condition for a clinical governance programme. Applying best practice in coronary heart disease requires a well-established infrastructure (good IT systems, disease registers), evidence-based protocols, monitoring systems, competent staff, multidisciplinary teamwork, etc.

Learning culture

Education and training programmes should be relevant to service needs whether at organisational or individual levels. Continuing professional development (CPD) programmes need to meet both the learning needs of individual health professionals and the wider service development needs of the NHS. You should no longer opt for CPD activities according to what you *want* to do, but rather according to what you *need* to do. Clinical governance underpins professional and service development.

> **Box 1.2**
>
> **Individual personal development plans**
> will feed into a
> **workplace- or practice-based personal and
> professional development plan**
> that will feed into
> **the primary care organisation's business plan**
> all of which are
> **underpinned by clinical governance.**[4]

Multidisciplinary learning will help the team to work closely to provide well co-ordinated multidisciplinary care.

Applying research and development in practice

The findings of the many thousands of research papers about cardio-vascular disease that are published in reputable journals each year are rarely applied in practice. This is because few health professionals or managers read such journals regularly, and consequently they are not aware of the research findings. Most practice teams do not have a system for reviewing important research papers and translating that review into practical action. The primary care organisation might help by relaying important new evidence to its constituent practices or to the general public. Agreement on local disease templates (e.g. for coronary heart disease) backed by resources should enable change to occur.

> **Box 1.3**
>
> Incorporating research-based evidence into everyday practice should promote policies on effective working, improve quality and contribute to a clinical governance culture.

Research increases our understanding of the causes and effects of coronary heart disease, as well as enabling the development of new treatments. However, it also sheds more light on how these treatments are applied in practice.

Box 1.4 Research continues to determine the role that homocysteine plays in vascular disease[5]

There is continuing uncertainty as to whether homocysteine is a cause of atherosclerosis or a marker for increased vascular risk. Over 30 cross-sectional and prospective studies involving more than 10 000 individuals have been performed. High plasma homocysteine levels induce vascular endothelial dysfunction. But we do not (yet?) have any evidence of benefits resulting from lowering homocysteine levels. Large-scale randomised placebo-controlled intervention trials are now under way.

Reliable and accurate data

Clinicians, patients and administrators need access to reliable and accurate data. Set the following standards for a general practice.

- Keep records in chronological order.
- Summarise medical records, within a specified time period for records of new patients.
- Review dates for checks on medication, with audit in place to monitor whether standards are adhered to and plan for under-performance if necessary.
- Use computers for diagnostic recording, and agree on Read codes for different coronary heart disease classifications as in Appendix 1.
- Record information from external sources (hospital, other organisations) that is relevant to individual patients or the practice.

Box 1.5

Read coding is the standard system of coding that is used in general practice. This is to be amalgamated with the system used by the College of American Pathologists to create a new coding system called SNOMED* clinical terms. It is expected that this new system will be available in late 2001 and will eventually replace the Read coding system. Any future transfer will be easier if medical records are already well ordered and classified.

* Systematised Nomenclature of Medicine.

Keep good written records of policies and audits that relate to coronary heart disease in the practice. An inspection at any time should show what audits have been undertaken and when, the changes in practice organisation that followed, the extent of staff training undertaken, and the future programme of monitoring.

There is still a great deal of resistance to full computerisation in practice teams. Ten ways to improve your practice team's enthusiasm for developing your IT infrastructure are listed in Box 1.6.

Box 1.6 10 ways to improve the likelihood of success with IT[6]

1 Start by considering your needs, not the technology.
2 Invest heavily in training for clinicians as well as IT staff.
3 Involve clinicians in all IT decisions.
4 Regard technology as a means to an end.
5 Use proper project management techniques.
6 Use the best IT staff you can afford.
7 Ensure that the IT solution delivers better patient care and clinical benefits.
8 Ensure that the suppliers deliver what is promised.
9 Adopt recommended solutions across the primary care organisation (PCO) to minimise compatibility problems.
10 Adopt a PCO-wide coding policy.

The Collection of Heart Data in General Practice (CHDGP) project has developed models for recording data in general practice on heart disease and related conditions, cerebrovascular disease and related conditions, hypertension, diabetes, asthma and severe mental illness.

The project is administered by Primary Care Information Services (PRIMIS), which is a training and support service structured to encourage best practice and development of information management skills in primary care. As part of that work, PRIMIS encourages individual practices to make use of data-entry templates that are self-designed or obtained from other bodies such as user groups. To help practices to compose their own templates, PRIMIS has compiled a query set to extract data from GP systems for analysis and feedback. This facility enables practices to build up a picture of CHD in their community. The specification of the query set is downloadable as an acrobat document from the PRIMIS website at:

http://www.primis.nhs.uk/documents/CHD_NSF_Specification_files/
CHD_NSF_Specification.pdf

Guidelines and instructions on implementing a data quality improvement scheme for coronary heart disease can be downloaded free from the following websites:

http://www.primis.nottingham.ac.uk/
http://www.nottingham.ac.uk/chdgp/guidelin.htm
http://www.nottingham.ac.uk/chdgp/handbook.htm

Well-managed resources and services

The things you need to achieve best practice should be in the right place at the right time, and working correctly every time.

Set standards in your practice or workplace for the following:

- access to premises and availability of services for people with special needs, such as those with disability from heart disease or stroke
- provision of routine and urgent appointments (e.g. for those with coronary heart disease)
- access to and provision for referral for investigation or treatment
- pro-active monitoring of chronic illness and disability
- alternatives to face-to-face consultations
- consultation length.

The primary care services to which the public requires access are information, advice, triage and treatment, continuity of care, personal care, emergency care and other services.

Systems should be designed to prevent and detect errors, so keep systems simple and sensible. Inform everyone how they operate so that they are less likely to bypass a system or make errors. Sort out good systems for the follow-up of patients with coronary heart disease and stroke.

There have been many protests about the introduction of the National Service Framework for Coronary Heart Disease in England without corresponding additional resources to enable its implementation. For instance, the Welsh Council of the Royal College of General Practitioners endorses the aims of the document, but has called for it to be realistic and operational and not purely aspirational, as described in Box 1.7.

Box 1.7 Welsh Council of the Royal College of General Practitioners' response to the National Service Framework for Coronary Heart Disease[7]

Whilst welcoming the document, recognising its importance and supporting its rationale, the Council feels that the document is unrealistic in terms of timescale and resource.
  Specifically:

- many issues are social and not health-related
- there are resource issues, involving both drugs and people; this will be a real test of whether resources follow extra workload – monitoring, use of statins, and anticoagulant clinics all have implications for primary care
- there are resource and staff implications for secondary care
- the document has been issued with no financial annex, therefore not identifying how much money will actually be filtered through to primary care
- there are queries about whether standards in the document actually represent legal standards and, if so, where that leaves GPs medico-legally
- the application of the criteria could cause more problems of access to general practitioners and to practice nurses
- some targets are aspirational and unrealistic.

Coherent teamwork

Teams do produce better patient care than single practitioners operating in a fragmented way. Effective teams make the most of the different contributions of individual clinical disciplines in delivering patient care. The characteristics of effective teams include the following:

- shared ownership of a common purpose
- clear goals for the contributions that each discipline makes
- open communication between team members
- opportunities for team members to enhance their skills.

The example in Box 1.8 demonstrates the power of teamwork that makes the most of new technology.

> **Box 1.8** Outreach cardiology service uses teleconferencing[8]
>
> The Hampstead group practice has developed a virtual outreach cardiology service jointly with a local hospital using a teleconferencing facility. Joint medical consultations occur involving the general practitioner, the consultant, the patient and practice nurses.

A team approach helps different team members to adopt an evidence-based approach to patient care – by having to justify their approach to the rest of the team.[9] The disciplines necessary for providing team-based coronary heart disease care include the GP and practice nurse, other community nurses, non-clinical staff, the dietitian and the community pharmacist, with help from other expert health professionals such as the cardiac specialist nurse, cardiac rehabilitation staff and the hospital-based cardiologist.

Meaningful involvement of patients and the public

Patients or carers, non-users of services, the local community, particular subgroups of the population or the general public will all have useful feedback and views. For example, ask for their views about the quality or type of healthcare on offer, planning future services, your systems, or how to locate services closer to the patient.

> **Box 1.9**
>
> The British Heart Foundation involves people suffering from cardiovascular problems in the preparation of their educative literature for patients, so that it is appropriate for such patients' needs and preferences.

The aims of user involvement and public participation include better outcomes of individual care and the health of the population, more locally responsive services and greater ownership of health services.[10] Those planning the services should develop a better understanding of why and how local services need to be changed. You might want to consult the public and health professionals about the closure of a community hospital, for example, without which those with chronic conditions such as coronary heart disease may have to travel further for their care.

Box 1.10 Coronary heart disease patient pathways[11]

A multi-agency group in North Stoke Primary Care Trust includes 'expert' patients in coronary heart disease. The group – termed the 'Zipper Club' – was set up in 1999. It has looked at how communication can be improved during the patient journey, and how patients can be empowered to work in partnership. Members of the group have mapped the different types of information for patients that exist (e.g. leaflets, videos, tapes and patient-held records). They found that there was a lack of communication and a duplication of effort, with patients' details being recorded many times over.

The Zipper Club has identified why communication is sometimes ineffective, and is introducing better information and advice for patients with coronary heart disease. Patient-held records are being trialled so that patients have copies of all test results and letters and can monitor their own progress.

Health gain

The two general approaches to improving health are the 'population' approach, which focuses on measures to improve health through the community, and the 'high-risk' approach, which focuses on vulnerable individuals who are at high risk of the condition or hazard.

The population strategy aims to shift the whole distribution of a risk factor in a favourable direction.[12] However, the 'prevention paradox' means that preventive actions that greatly benefit the population at large may bring only small benefits for individuals.

Box 1.11

Changing the population distribution of a risk factor is better than targeting people who are at high risk.[12]

The high-risk approach aims to detect people at high risk of disease and to lower their risk by treatment. We generally use a targeted approach in primary care to identify people who are at risk or whose coronary heart disease is currently undiagnosed, rather than using a population-based approach.

The two approaches are not mutually exclusive, and they often need to be combined with legislation and community action. Health goals include the following:

- a good quality of life
- avoiding premature death
- equal opportunities for health.

Cigarette smoking, hypertension, diabetes, age, raised total cholesterol and low levels of high-density lipoproteins are major and independent risk factors for coronary heart disease.

Modifiable risk factors include the following:

- obesity
- lack of exercise
- smoking
- high lipid levels.

These are associated with potential health gains by reducing the risks of coronary heart disease in those people who have diabetes. Modifying these risk factors will usually require several different interventions per individual, in order to optimise control of blood pressure and plasma lipids and help patients to lose weight and stop smoking.

Confidentiality

Confidentiality is a component of clinical governance that is often overlooked. Experienced health professionals and managers may assume that junior or new staff know all about confidentiality, and of course they may not. There are many difficult situations in the NHS where one person asks for information about another's medical condition. For example, it is not always obvious whether test results should be given to or withheld from someone else enquiring on their behalf if the patient is vulnerable in some way (e.g. affected by a severe stroke).

The Caldicott Committee Report describes the following principles of good practice to safeguard confidentiality when information is being used for non-clinical purposes.[13]

- Justify the purpose.
- Do not use patient-identifiable information unless it is absolutely necessary to do so.
- Use the minimum necessary patient-identifiable information.

- Access to patient-identifiable information should be on a strict need-to-know basis.
- Everyone with access to patient-identifiable information should be aware of his or her responsibilities.

Evidence-based culture – policy and practice

The key features of whether or not local guidelines worked in one initiative[14] were as follows.

- There was multidisciplinary involvement in drawing them up.
- A systematic review of the literature underpinned the guidelines, with graded recommendations for best practice linked to the evidence.
- There was ownership at national and local levels.
- A local implementation plan ensured that the need for resources, time, staff, education and training was foreseen, met and supported.
- Plans were made to sustain the guidelines – which were user friendly, and could be modified to suit individual practitioners and patients.

There are several systems of grading evidence. A classification[15] that is often quoted gives the strength of evidence as shown in Box 1.12.

Box 1.12 Strength of evidence

Type I:　strong evidence from at least one systematic review of multiple well-designed randomised controlled trials (RCTs).

Type II:　strong evidence from at least one properly designed randomised controlled trial of appropriate size.

Type III:　evidence from well-designed trials without randomisation, single group pre–post, cohort, time-series or matched case–control studies.

Type IV:　evidence from well-designed non-experimental studies from more than one centre or research group.

Type V:　opinions of respected authorities, based on clinical evidence, descriptive studies or reports of expert committees.

Other categories of evidence are listed in the compendium of the best available evidence for effective healthcare, *Clinical Evidence*, which is updated every six months. This categorisation of evidence is perhaps more useful to the health professional in everyday work.[16]

Box 1.13

Beneficial:	interventions whose effectiveness has been shown by clear evidence from controlled trials.
Likely to be beneficial:	interventions for which effectiveness is less well established than for those listed under 'beneficial'.
Trade-off between benefits and harm:	interventions for which clinicians and patients should weigh up the beneficial and harmful effects according to individual circumstances and priorities.
Unknown effectiveness:	interventions for which there are currently insufficient data or data of inadequate quality (this includes interventions that are widely accepted as beneficial but which have never been formally tested in randomised control trials (RCTs), often because RCTs would be regarded as unethical).
Unlikely to be beneficial:	interventions for which lack of effectiveness is less well established than for those listed under 'likely to be ineffective or harmful'.
Likely to be ineffective or harmful:	interventions whose ineffectiveness or harmfulness has been demonstrated by clear evidence.

The Scottish Intercollegiate Guidelines Network (SIGN) has produced over 50 evidence-based guidelines. They base their recommendations on systematic reviews of the scientific literature. SIGN takes the view that guidelines do not provide answers to every clinical question, nor do they guarantee a successful outcome in all cases. Rather, the ultimate decision about a particular clinical procedure or treatment will depend on clinical judgement and each individual patient's condition, circumstances and preferences.[17] SIGN sees local ownership of the implementation of guidelines as crucial to success in changing practice. There are SIGN guidelines for *Lipids and the Primary Prevention of Coronary Heart Disease*[18] and *Secondary Prevention of Coronary Heart Disease Following Myocardial Infarction.*[19]

Accountability and performance

Health professionals may not always realise that they are accountable to others from outside their own professions, especially if they have self-employed status, as do GPs, pharmacists and optometrists. However, in fact they are accountable to the following:

* the general public
* the profession – to maintain standards of knowledge and skills of the profession as a whole
* the government – and employer – who expect high standards of healthcare from the workforce.

Identify and rectify under-performance at an early stage by, for example:

* regular appraisals (at least annually) linked to clinical governance and personal development plans – appraisals should be supportive meetings, but need a mechanism for dealing with under-performance if it crops up
* detecting those who have significant health problems and referring them for help
* systematic audit that distinguishes individuals' performance from the overall performance of the practice team
* an open learning culture in which team members are discouraged from covering up colleagues' inadequacies so that problems can be resolved at an early stage.

Clinicians may see the performance assessment framework as a management tool that is not particularly relevant to their clinical practice. However, it does reinforce a clinical governance culture whereby good clinical management and organisational management have a symbiotic relationship.

Box 1.14

The NHS performance assessment framework has six components, namely health improvement, fair access, efficiency, effective delivery of appropriate care, user/carer experience and health outcomes.

Health promotion

People with coronary heart disease will benefit if they are well informed about their condition and able to participate in making decisions about the management of their condition. Good information will help patients with coronary heart disease to make choices about their diet, smoking, physical activity and other health-related behaviour.

Box 1.15

Smoking cessation services have been targeted at the 26 Health Action Zones in England and their disadvantaged populations. Most of them have concentrated on young people and pregnant women as priority groups, in order to limit the harmful effects of smoking on future generations.[20]

Audit and evaluation

Audit will probably be the method you think of first for finding out how well you are doing and what it is you need to learn.

Box 1.16 Audit reveals unequal treatment for elderly people with heart failure[21]

A review of the case-notes of 583 people with heart failure showed that older men and women were less likely to have undergone echocardiography or to have received an angiotensin-converting-enzyme (ACE) inhibitor than younger people. There were no statistically significant differences between the sexes when women's disproportionately older age was allowed for.

You might look at the extent to which you are adhering to practice protocols – for instance, whether you are giving consistent advice to everyone with risks of cardiovascular disease and/or diabetes about smoking habits, weight and exercise.

> **Box 1.17** 'From one patient, through clinical audit, needs assessment and commissioning into quality improvement'[22]
>
> A significant event as part of an audit cycle can make a real impact on improvement of the quality of care. A 52-year-old patient's death from an acute myocardial infarction was reviewed by the practice team. They looked back at how they had managed his multiple risk factors over the preceding 10 years – his hypertension, hyperlipidaemia and overweight. They reviewed the literature and the practice protocols. Then they examined how well they were operating primary and secondary prevention of ischaemic heart disease for adults registered with the practice. They revised the practice protocol to take a more aggressive and proactive approach to hyperlipidaemia. The practice allocated money to cover the additional drug costs from their then fundholding budget. The audit of the case study led to changes in the practice organisation and clinical practice that improved the quality of care for those with risk factors for heart disease.

Core requirements

You cannot deliver clinical governance without well-trained and competent staff, the right skill mix of staff, and a safe and comfortable working environment.

There is accumulating evidence that management of coronary heart disease according to best practice is cost-effective, but research is still needed on the relative cost-effectiveness of different methods of screening.

The NHS Plan for England[23] describes the core requirements for the NHS which are part of a clinical governance culture in relation to the following:

- partnership – working together across the NHS to ensure the best possible care
- performance – acting to review and deliver higher standards of healthcare
- the professions and wider workforce – breaking down barriers between different disciplines (e.g. through multidisciplinary teamwork between GPs and nurses with pharmacists and other independent contractors)

- patient care – access, convenient services, and empowerment to take a full part in decision making about their own medical care and in planning and providing health services in general
- prevention – promoting healthy living across all sections of society and tackling variations in care.

Box 1.18 Structured care of patients known to have ischaemic heart disease through a nurse-led clinic[8]

All patients who were identified as having ischaemic heart disease in one practice were invited to a structured clinical assessment by nurses with specialised training. Care was provided through an evidence-based protocol. A re-audit of the project showed improvements in care.

Risk management

People may underestimate relative risks as applied to themselves and their own behaviour. For example, many smokers accept the relationship between smoking tobacco and disease, but do not believe that they personally are at risk. People usually have a reasonable idea of the *relative risks* of various activities and behaviours, although their personal estimates of the *magnitude* of the risks tend to be biased, small probabilities often being overestimated and high probabilities often being underestimated.[3]

Risk management in general practice mainly centres on assessing probabilities that potential or actual hazards will give rise to harm. Consider how bad the risk is, how likely the risk is, when the risk will happen, if ever, and how certain you are of estimates about the risks. This applies just as much whether the risk is an environmental or organisational risk in the practice or a clinical risk.

Good practice means understanding and managing risk – both clinical and organisational aspects. Undertaking audit more systematically will reduce the risks of omission. Common areas of risk in providing healthcare services include the following:[3]

- out-of-date clinical practice
- lack of continuity of care
- poor communication
- mistakes in patient care
- patient complaints
- financial risk – insufficient resources

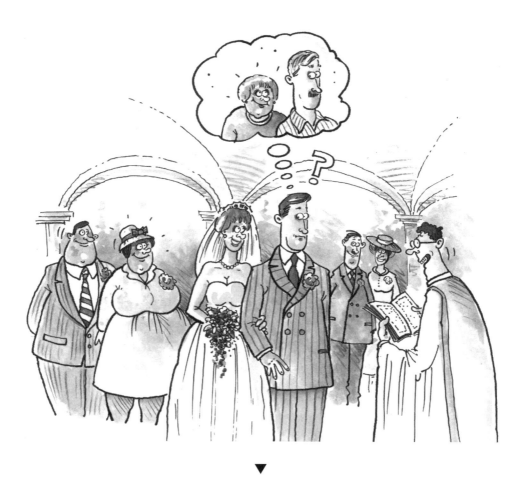

Relative risks!

- reputation
- staff morale.

Communicating and managing risks on an individual basis with patients depends on finding ways to explain risks and elicit people's values and preferences. They can then make decisions themselves to take risks or choose between alternatives that involve different risks and benefits.

Having a system for gathering patients' comments or a good patient complaint system should reduce the risk of a recurrence of the event which originally triggered the complaint.

Reflection exercise

Exercise 1

Review and plan your clinical management of coronary heart disease.

Think how you might integrate the 14 components of clinical governance into your personal development plan or your practice personal and professional development plan. Examples are given for each component listed below. Complete this yourself from your own perspective.

- *Establishing a learning culture*: e.g. informal discussion about hypertension guidelines between GPs, nurses and the community pharmacist.
- *Managing resources and services*: e.g. review the roles and responsibilities for managing post-myocardial infarction care by members of the practice team and attached staff.
- *Establishing a research and development culture*: e.g. share findings in key research papers on best practice for managing heart failure or stroke among the practice team members.
- *Reliable and accurate data*: e.g. keep electronic records (both individual and team) so that everyone uses the same Read codes (or SNOMED; *see* page 6) and enters data consistently. Any audit exercises can be repeated next year and the results compared.
- *Evidence-based practice and policy*: e.g. update the evidence-based protocol for managing hyperlipidaemia.
- *Confidentiality:* e.g. check that everyone is adhering to your agreed code of practice for giving results or advice at the reception desk.

- *Health gain*: e.g. target those with diabetes for particular efforts in reducing their risk factors for coronary heart disease.
- *Coherent team*: e.g. communicate new systems for classifying smoking status to the rest of your practice team.
- *Audit and evaluation*: e.g. undertake a significant event audit and act on the findings to improve the quality of aspects of coronary heart disease care.
- *Meaningful involvement of patients and the public*: e.g. listen to and act on the comments about the care and services you are providing that are made by those who have had strokes.
- *Health promotion:* e.g. obtain or write literature promoting physical activity through local walks.
- *Risk management:* e.g. establish systems and procedures to identify, analyse and control clinical risks such as those from poor repeat-prescribing practices.
- *Accountability and performance*: e.g. keep good records of those who have had a myocardial infarction, to demonstrate best practice in cardiac rehabilitation.
- *Core requirements*: e.g. agree roles and responsibilities within the practice team, such as nurse referral to GPs, and train receptionists to act in a crisis situation.

Now that you have completed this interactive reflection exercise, transfer the information to the empty template of the personal development plan on pages 142–151 if you are working on your own learning plan, or to the practice personal and professional development plan on pages 165–172 if you are working on a practice team learning plan. Don't forget to keep the evidence of your learning in your personal portfolio.

References

1 Lilley R (1999) *Making Sense of Clinical Governance*. Radcliffe Medical Press, Oxford.
2 Chambers R and Wakley G (2000) *Making Clinical Governance Work for You*. Radcliffe Medical Press, Oxford.
3 Mohanna K and Chambers R (2001) *Risk Matters: communicating risk, clinical risk management*. Radcliffe Medical Press, Oxford.
4 Wakley G, Chambers R and Field S (2000) *Continuing Professional Development: making it happen*. Radcliffe Medical Press, Oxford.

5 Chambers J, Seddon M, Shah S *et al.* (2001) Homocysteine – a novel risk factor for vascular disease. *J R Soc Med.* **94**: 10–13.

6 Gillies A (2000) *Information and IT for Primary Care.* Radcliffe Medical Press, Oxford.

7 Royal College of General Practitioners of Wales (2001) *Report for UK Council January Meeting.* Royal College of General Practitioners, London.

8 NHS Beacon Services (2000) *NHS Beacons Learning Handbook 2000/2001. Volume 1.* NHS Beacons Services, Petersfield.

9 Miller C, Ross N and Freeman M (1999) *Shared Learning and Clinical Teamwork: new directions in education and multiprofessional practice.* The English National Board for Nursing, Midwifery and Health Visiting, University of Brighton, Brighton.

10 Chambers R (2000) *Involving Patients and the Public: how to do it better.* Radcliffe Medical Press, Oxford.

11 Parkinson P (2001) *CHD Patient Pathways.* North Stoke Primary Care Trust, Stoke-on-Trent.

12 Hofman A and Vandenbroucke JP (1992) Geoffrey Rose's big idea. Changing the population distribution of a risk factor is better than targeting people at high risk. *BMJ.* **305**: 1519–20.

13 Department of Health (1997) Report of the review of patient-identifiable information. In: *The Caldicott Committee Report.* Department of Health, London.

14 Donald P (2000) Promoting local ownership of guidelines. *Guidelines Pract.* **3**: 17.

15 Muir Gray JA (1997) *Evidence-Based Healthcare.* Churchill Livingstone, Edinburgh.

16 Barton S (ed.) (2001) *Clinical Evidence. Issue 5.* BMJ Publishing Group, London.

17 Royal College of General Practitioners (Scotland), Scottish Heart and Arterial Disease Risk Prevention and the Scottish Intercollegiate Guidelines Network (2000) *The Heart Pack: coronary heart disease resource directory.* Royal College of General Practitioners, Edinburgh.

18 Scottish Intercollegiate Guidelines Network (1999) *Lipids and the Primary Prevention of Coronary Heart Disease.* SIGN Secretariat, Edinburgh.

19 Scottish Intercollegiate Guidelines Network (2000) *Secondary Prevention of Coronary Heart Disease following Myocardial Infarction.* SIGN Secretariat, Edinburgh.

20 Department of Health (2000) *Statistics on Smoking Cessation Services in Health Action Zones: England, April 1999 to March 2000.* Statistical Press Release. Department of Health, London.

21 Hood S, Taylor S, Roeves A *et al.* (2000) Are there age and sex differences in the investigation and treatment of heart failure? A population-based study. *Br J Gen Pract.* **50**: 559–63.

22 Pringle M (1998) Preventing ischaemic heart disease in one general practice: from one patient, through clinical audit, needs assessment, and commissioning into quality improvement. *BMJ.* **317**: 1120–24.

23 Department of Health (2000) *The NHS Plan for England.* DoH, London.

CHAPTER 2

Hypertension

What is hypertension?

That's a really difficult question – it depends on who you ask! Blood pressure is the hydrostatic pressure that the blood exerts on the vessel walls. When we measure the blood pressure and call it 'hypertension', we are taking a decision about the harmful effects of a surrogate marker. That is, the decisions are being taken about something that we *can* measure with regard to something that we *cannot* measure, namely the risk that the blood vessels or the heart are diseased or will become damaged.

Therefore other indicators of risk of damage to the cardiovascular system have to be taken into consideration when deciding when the measured blood pressure is too high or 'hypertensive'. If you do not think of hypertension as a disease, but as a risk measurement for other diseases, then it becomes easier to understand why there are so many definitions and variations. It all depends on the disease you are considering and the other risk factors that are present.

Definitions of 'hypertension' vary according to the country and population,[1] and have changed over time. The *British Hypertension Society Guidelines*[2] and the *National Service Framework for Coronary Heart Disease*[3] define hypertension as:

> 'a sustained systolic blood pressure of 140 mmHg or more, or a diastolic blood pressure of 85 mmHg or more'.

Systolic and diastolic pressures are continuously related to the risk of developing cardiovascular disease, and the risk extends into the range usually regarded as 'normal' blood pressures.

The same publications[1–3] recommend *treatment* for people who have:

> 'sustained systolic blood pressure of 160 mmHg or more and/or diastolic pressure of 100 mmHg or more',

and treatment at lower limits for those who have other risk factors:

> 'sustained systolic pressure of 140–159 mmHg or diastolic pressure of 85–89 mmHg'.

Other risk factors include the following:

- evidence of established cardiovascular disease
- diabetes
- a 10-year risk of cardiovascular disease of more than 15% (*see* later in this chapter for an account of the use of coronary heart risk charts or computer programs)
- the presence of target organ damage.

Health professionals should be very careful not to alarm patients unnecessarily about the potential risks from hypertension before a series of blood pressure checks over time has established that there is indeed a hypertensive problem.

Measuring blood pressure

Measure blood pressure in adults every five years.[2] Those with high normal pressures and no other risk factors (135–139 mmHg systolic and/or 85–89 mmHg diastolic) or with a previously recorded high level should have an annual recording.

Box 2.1

A recent review published in the *British Medical Journal* concluded that, too often, accuracy of blood pressure measuring devices had been sacrificed for technological ingenuity. The article emphasised the variability in blood pressure measurements between manual sphygmomanometers, self-measurement blood pressure devices automated for upper arm and wrist use, specialised clinical blood pressure measuring equipment and ambulatory measurement recorders – all made by different manufacturers. The authors urged that all blood pressure devices should be independently validated against specific systolic and diastolic blood pressures.[4]

Traditionally, blood pressure has been measured in millimetres of mercury (mmHg) with a mercury sphygmomanometer. Attempts

Table 2.1 Korotkov sounds and phases*

Phase	Sound
Phase 1	Onset of sharp and clear sounds; gives the systolic pressure
Phases 2 and 3	Blowing or swishing, but still quite clear as the pressure is falling. Occasionally absent – the silence replacing them is termed the 'auscultatory gap'
Phase 4	Muffled fading sound; sometimes given as the diastolic pressure, especially if it continues to zero; specify if used
Phase 5	No sound; correlates better with intra-arterial pressure; preferred phase for diastolic pressure recording[2]

* In most people, phases 4 and 5 are within 10 mmHg of each other, but it is a good habit to record which is used in individual patients in order to reduce inter-observer error.

have been made to change this to standard international units (SI), where 100 mmHg = 13.3 kPa (a kiloPascal is the measurement used for pressure), but this transition has so far been unsuccessful in clinical practice. The Korotkov sounds have been used to determine the systolic and diastolic pressures by auscultation with a stethoscope over (usually) the brachial artery. The Korotkov sounds are divided into five phases (*see* Table 2.1).

Aneroid sphygmomanometers work on a bellows system and give similar readings to mercury devices, but are slightly more prone to error, so check them against another machine every 6 months. The best device for reducing error from the machine and user is a correctly calibrated electronic device used over the upper arm with a suitable size of cuff to measure the pressure in the brachial artery. The use of mercury sphygmomanometers should be phased out to avoid the dangers of mercury spillage and to comply with European Commission directives.

Errors arise in any measurement. Sources of error in blood pressure recording are shown in Box 2.2.

Box 2.2 Potential errors when recording blood pressure

Measuring device	Poor maintenance	• Blocked vent on mercury column • Faulty valves on inflation cuff • Not recently re-calibrated (especially aneroid or electronic)
Measuring device	Poor design or use	• Wrist or finger devices • If mercury column – long tubes or height above or below patient • Mercury scale not upright
Cuff	Incorrectly applied	• Clothing pushed up to constrict arm above cuff • Centre of bladder not over artery
Cuff	Incorrect size	• Use an appropriate size for the limb – bladder of cuff should encircle arm
Position of the patient	Arm	• Should be supported as muscle tension increases the diastolic pressure • Should be horizontal at the level of the fourth intercostal space at the sternum (raising or lowering the arm may make a difference of as much as 10 mmHg) • Pressures can vary between the right and left arm (record which one is used) • Arm should be at rest when recording – you may need to hold the wrist to avoid the patient waving their hand while talking!
State of the patient	Anxiety, pain, full bladder, exercise, eating, smoking, alcohol	• Anxiety or pain are difficult to avoid, but record them for later comparison • Eating, smoking and alcohol consumption are best avoided for at least 30 minutes before recording • Allow the patient to empty their bladder before recording • Rest for 5 minutes before recording
Environment	Noise, temperature, etc.	• May affect the concentration of the observer and the state of the patient

Recording	Observer bias	• Seeing previous readings, or an expectation that the level will be normal or raised
Recording	Digit preference	• Many people who are reading a scale will approximate (e.g. give a reading of '5' despite the fact that the scale is marked in 2 mmHg graduations)
Recording	Lack of concentration	• Especially when the observer is rushed
Recording	Hearing loss	• Use an electronic device, not a stethoscope
Recording	Visual problems	• Make sure that the scale or reading can be seen clearly
Recording	Inaccurate	• We all write things down wrongly sometimes

Given the potential for error, do not rely on a single measurement of a raised level. The criteria for treatment is for *sustained* hypertension. Use two measurements at each of several visits. You may want to use ambulatory blood pressure recording if:

- you suspect 'white-coat hypertension'
- there is considerable variation in the recordings made at each visit
- treatment is failing
- symptoms suggest episodes of hypotension.

'White-coat hypertension' – that is the tendency to have an elevated blood pressure whilst under mild stress (e.g. from consulting a doctor or nurse) – affects about 10% of the population. It may indicate an increased risk of left ventricular hypertrophy.[5]

You will want to use the blood pressure measurements for audit purposes, so give some thought to how and where the values are recorded. Most computer systems have dedicated areas or boxes for entry. Train everyone to enter the values here, rather than recording them in free text. They cannot be retrieved from free text, and it will look as if you have not taken the measurements. If you are still using a paper-based system, make sure that the values can be retrieved easily and consistently – perhaps by using a stamp, a different colour of ink or a separate chart insert.

Initial assessment of the patient with hypertension

Do you already have guidelines? Check that they are up to date and accessible to all clinical staff. The British Hypertension Society guidelines appear in the publication, *Guidelines*,[6] or on the *e*Guidelines website (*see* Appendix 3).

You will want to establish the following:

* whether the patient has an underlying cause for hypertension (*see* Table 2.2)

Table 2.2 Is there an underlying cause for the hypertension?

Cause	*What to look for*
Drug-induced	Medication such as non-steroidal anti-inflammatory drugs, corticosteroids, combined oral contraceptives, cyclosporin, erythropoietin
Endocrine	
Primary aldosteronism	Tetany, muscle weakness, polyuria, hypokalaemia
Cushing's syndrome	Truncal obesity, striae, etc.
Phaeochromocytoma	Intermittent high blood pressure, sweating attacks, palpitations
Acromegaly	Enlargement of the hands and feet, coarsening of facial features, visual field loss, etc.
Vascular	
Coarctation of aorta	Delayed or weak femoral pulses
Renal artery stenosis	Peripheral vascular disease, abdominal bruit
Renal	
Chronic pyelonephritis	History of recurrent infections
Diabetic nephropathy	Microalbuminuria or proteinuria
Glomerulonephritis	Microscopic haematuria
Obstructive uropathy	Abdominal or flank mass
Polycystic kidneys	Abdominal or flank mass, microscopic haematuria, family history
Connective tissue disorders	Symptoms or signs of scleroderma, systemic lupus erythematosus, polyarteritis nodosa, retroperitoneal fibrosis.

- what other risk factors are present (smoking, obesity, diabetes, etc.)
- any complications that are already present (e.g. previous stroke)
- if there is any end-organ damage (e.g. left ventricular hypertrophy)
- if there are any other conditions that might affect treatment (e.g. asthma preventing the use of beta-blocker drugs).

History and examination will reveal most of these factors. Investigations that can be performed routinely include the following:

- urine strip test for blood and protein
- blood electrolytes and creatinine
- blood glucose
- ratio of serum total:HDL cholesterol
- electrocardiogram.

You will need to refer some patients for specialist opinion, for the following reasons:

- specialist investigations
- very high levels of blood pressure (more than 220/120 mmHg), accelerated increases (malignant hypertension) or impending complications
- treatment difficulties
- special problems (e.g. unusually variable levels or pregnancy).

Management of established hypertension

You could encourage lifestyle interventions (*see* Box 2.3) in patients who have mild hypertension but no target organ damage or cardiovascular complications, and reassess them after 4–6 months. Introduce these interventions at the same time in patients when drug treatment is indicated. Evidence about changing behaviour[7] shows that it *is* worth making the effort to advise people about lifestyle changes. Such changes can make a substantial impact on risk factors, and even small changes in weight can reduce blood pressure readings – blood pressure falls by 2.5/1.5 mmHg for each kilogram of weight lost.

Box 2.3 Non-drug treatments[2]

To lower blood pressure
Weight reduction
Dynamic exercise such as brisk walking (rather than isometric exercise such as weight training)

Limiting alcohol intake to < 22 units in men or < 15 units in women per week

Reducing *added* salt in the diet, or avoiding salty foods

Increasing intake of fruit and vegetables to at least five portions daily

Reducing salt content of the diet

To reduce the risk of cardiovascular disease

Stopping smoking

Reducing saturated fat content of the diet, and replacing it with polyunsaturated or monounsaturated fat

Increasing intake of oily fish

The hypertension optimal treatment (HOT) trial[2] suggested that the optimal blood pressure for reduction of cardiovascular events was 139/83 mmHg. The numbers in this trial were not large, and there were no obvious disadvantages in the group whose blood pressure was below 150/90 mmHg. Patients with diabetes had greater lowering of their risk if their diastolic blood pressure was kept below 80 mmHg. Discuss the optimal treatment with each patient, as not everyone will be willing or able to achieve these targets.

Antihypertensive drug therapy

The British Hypertension Society guidelines recommend starting drug treatment in people who have a sustained systolic pressure of 160 mmHg or more, or a sustained diastolic pressure of 100 mmHg or more[2] (*see* Figure 2.1 – this algorithm does not describe some of the lower treatment thresholds with co-morbidities given in other guidelines – *see* p. 37 for instance).

Three long-term, double-blind studies compared the major classes of antihypertensive drugs and found no consistent or important differences in efficacy, side-effects or quality of life.[2] There were differences between the classes of drugs related to ethnic group and age. Treatment trials with beta-blocker or thiazide drugs provide most of the evidence about the benefits of blood pressure lowering for reducing cardiovascular risk. Consider individual patient variation when deciding which treatment to choose (*see* Table 2.3).

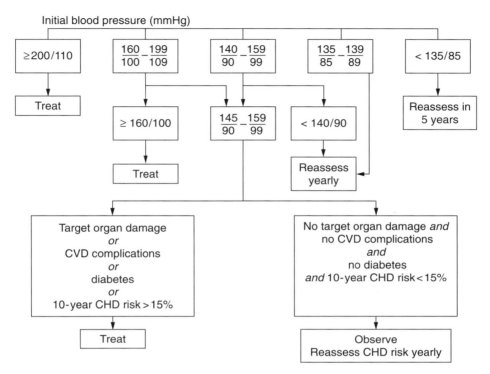

Figure 2.1: Flow diagram for antihypertensive drug therapy and cardiac risk.[2,6]

Tailor the drug regime to suit the patient whenever possible. If there are no indications to direct the first choice to specific drugs, then a low dose of a thiazide (e.g. bendrofluazide 2.5 mg or hydrochlorothiazide 25 mg) is cost-effective. The dose–response curve for thiazides shows that increasing the dose does not increase efficacy, so change the type of medication, or add in another, if there is a poor response.

Unless it is very urgent, only change the therapy after an interval of about 4 weeks. Always check first that the patient is taking the medication. Important concepts include the following.

- *Partnership*: successful treatment depends on partnerships between the patients and healthcare professionals.
- *Empowerment*: our role is to help to empower those with hypertension to find the best ways of helping themselves to modify their lifestyles.
- *Judgement*: beware of imposing your views – the people with hypertension are the ones who really understand their experiences and problems.

Table 2.3 Major classes of drugs for treatment of patients with hypertension, derived from the British Hypertension Society guidelines[2,6]

Class of drug	Other conditions from which the patient is suffering			
	Drug of choice	Possible choice	Caution	Contraindication
Thiazide	Elderly	Good initial choice for most	Abnormal lipids	Gout
Beta-blockers	Myocardial infarction, angina	Heart failure*	Heart failure, abnormal lipids, peripheral vascular disease	Asthma, chronic obstructive pulmonary disease, heart block
Angiotensin-converting-enzyme (ACE) inhibitors	Heart failure, left ventricular dysfunction, type I diabetic nephropathy	Chronic renal disease,* type II diabetic nephropathy	Peripheral vascular disease (exclude renovascular disease)	Pregnancy, renovascular disease
Angiotensin-II receptor antagonists	As for ACE inhibitors, but preferable if cough develops with ACE treatment	Intolerance to other antihypertensive drugs	As for ACE inhibitors	As for ACE inhibitors
Alpha-blockers	Prostatism	Abnormal lipids	Postural hypotension	Urinary incontinence
Calcium-channel antagonists (dihydropyridine; class II)	Isolated systolic hypertension in the elderly	Angina, elderly African-Caribbean	Headache, flushing, oedema	
Calcium-channel antagonists (rate limiting; class I and III)	Angina	Myocardial infarction	Combination with beta-blocker	Heart block, heart failure

* But may worsen, seek specialist advice.

- *Values*: people's values and priorities change with time. They may be quite different to your current values, but no less valid.
- *Autonomy*: autonomy should be a fundamental right for everyone. Having to take treatment and attend for check-ups means a loss of some aspects of autonomy.
- *Listening*: active non-judgemental listening is the core art of medicine and healthcare, and is crucial to gaining an understanding of people with hypertension.
- *Shared decision making:* people with chronic conditions need to be able to take their own decisions about their management, based on the expert information communicated to them by health professionals. Shared decision making leads to concordance.
- *Concordance:* a negotiated agreement about treatment between the patient and the healthcare professional[8,9] allows patients to take informed decisions on the degree of risk or suffering that they themselves are willing to accept. In contrast, 'compliance' with treatment or lifestyle changes implies that the patient follows instructions from health professionals to a greater or lesser degree.

Try to give as few drugs as possible, and preferably in a single daily dose. It is really difficult to remember to do something new every day, let alone several times a day. If the hypertension is not severe, but is not controlled on the first drug, change the medication and check again after 4 weeks. If the levels are more severely raised, add in therapy in a stepwise manner – you can always drop drugs again once the levels are under control. Most patients seem to require more than one anti-hypertensive drug.[2]

Two drugs at lower dosages often work better than a large dose of a single one, and have fewer side-effects. Suitable combinations of drugs might include the following:

- a thiazide and a beta-blocker, such as atenolol
- a thiazide with an ACE inhibitor
- a beta-blocker with a calcium-channel antagonist (dihydropyridine type)
- a calcium-channel antagonist with an ACE inhibitor.

Obviously you should avoid a combination of a beta-blocker and a rate-limiting calcium-channel antagonist! Other combinations to avoid are an ACE inhibitor and an angiotensin II antagonist, or an ACE inhibitor with a potassium-sparing diuretic. Commonly used third-line combinations of drugs include the following:

- a diuretic with an ACE inhibitor and a calcium antagonist
- a diuretic with a beta-blocker and a calcium antagonist.

Fixed-dose combinations may be sensible and convenient once the patient is happy with the medication and is well controlled, provided that there are no major cost implications. Beware of unfamiliar drug combinations that may contain the same class of drug as is already being prescribed singly.

Box 2.4

Mr A came across as an intimidating new patient who talked condescendingly about his 'good friend John', one of the local cardiologists, who had started him on his medication. He implied that his poorly controlled blood pressure readings were the fault of the doctor, and asked when the equipment had last been checked for accuracy. The doctor suggested adding in verapamil to the new ACE inhibitor that he thought the patient was taking. He was embarrassed to find that the medication which the patient was taking was a combination drug that included verapamil and an ACE inhibitor, and not one of the newer ACE inhibitors alone, as he had thought.

The PRODIGY guidelines (*see* websites in Appendix 3) on hypertension contain detailed lists of the recommended medication for treatment of hypertension. The most cost-effective drugs for which there is good evidence are cited. The guidelines give some useful scenarios that you could use for small group discussion and learning about the management of hypertension. You may want to refine the recommendations to suit your own practice or local guidelines.

Follow-up management

Once stabilised, patients are usually reviewed every 3 to 6 months, and the urine is tested for protein and blood every year. If patients are on diuretics or ACE-inhibitor drugs, check electrolytes and renal function every year as well. Reconsider the cardiac risk factors at the annual check-up.

You may want to establish or revise the practice protocol for the follow-up of patients. Practice nurses often manage the follow-up, with referral of the patient to the doctor if blood pressure levels are not controlled. Consider carefully how you will introduce any changes and the implications for workload and training.

A paper published in 2000 from 27 general practices in Avon[10] compared outcomes in practices randomised to use a computer-based clinical decision support system plus a risk chart, the risk chart alone, or usual care. Neither the 'computer system' nor the 'chart alone' reduced cardiovascular risk. The patients in the 'chart alone' group showed a significant reduction in systolic blood pressure and increased prescriptions of cardiovascular drugs. The authors suggested that the 'computer system' may have distracted health professionals, and that such systems need careful evaluation before being introduced into routine primary care. The study highlights the need to offer training to people who will be using previously unfamiliar tools – enthusiasm from the innovators is not enough!

Estimation and prevention of cardiac risk

The Framingham risk score is available in an easy-to-use pro forma on *e*MIMS (free discs are sent with the monthly *MIMS* publication, or see the list of websites in Appendix 3). It can be used to predict the 10-year absolute risk of a coronary heart disease event. It is only useful for those who do not currently have any evidence of established vascular disease. Patients with an absolute risk of more than 15% should have their hypertension controlled to achieve the target levels, and should take statins if necessary to lower the total cholesterol concentration to below 5 mmol/L.

The Sheffield table[6] helps with decision making about the various factors to take into consideration when deciding on added treatment. It is also available on *e*Guidelines (*see* list of websites in Appendix 3). It gives the cholesterol concentration at ages 30 to 70 years in 2-year bands, separately for men and women, calculated together with the added risks of hypertension, left ventricular hypertrophy (if hypertensive), smoking or diabetes. The table can be used to predict the need for measurement or treatment at an older age. It is not useful for secondary prevention of coronary heart disease when treatment with a statin for a raised cholesterol level is indicated in any case. The table may underestimate the risks in UK Asians, people with low HDL cholesterol levels, and those with a strong family history of premature coronary heart disease or familial hyperlipidaemia.

Give aspirin, 75 mg daily, to patients who have established cardiovascular disease, or who are at high risk according to either of the two measures above, or the British Societies 'Cardiac Risk Assessor' computer program or poster charts (available from the British Heart Foundation; *see* list of useful addresses in Appendix 3 or in a reduced form in the *Guidelines*[6] publication). Trials have not justified the use of aspirin in patients with uncomplicated hypertension who are aged under 50 years.[2]

Tailoring your treatment for special categories of patient

Tailor your treatment to the individual characteristics and needs of the patient.

Box 2.5

Mr L was a keen marathon runner. He was amazed when he was told that he had a raised blood pressure, and was very disappointed when it did not settle on repeated measurement. He resisted the doctor's offer of drug treatment for some time, instead trying biofeedback, with salt restriction and home monitoring. He already had little body fat, a diet containing plenty of vegetables and fruit, was a non-smoker and certainly had plenty of exercise. Eventually he accepted that he needed to reduce the level of his blood pressure. He looked up all of the side-effects of the drugs available, and discussed with his doctor which ones would be least likely to affect his marathon running. He did not wish to take thiazides (due to their effect on potassium levels) or beta-blockers (due to heart rate limitation by these drugs), which the practice had recommended as the preferred starting medication. He agreed to try an ACE inhibitor, but needed considerable support for his many psychosomatic side-effects until he settled.

Ethnic groups

Patients of Asian origin living in the UK who have hypertension are more at risk of diabetes and coronary artery disease. Thiazides should be used with caution, as they can worsen glucose intolerance. Patients of African-Caribbean origin seem to respond less well to beta-blockers and ACE-inhibitor drugs, and better blood pressure control is achieved on thiazide and calcium-channel antagonists.[11]

Older people with hypertension

Hypertension, especially isolated systolic hypertension (160 mmHg systolic pressure or more, with a diastolic pressure of less than 90 mmHg), is found in more than 50% of those over 60 years of age. Cardiovascular risks are higher in patients with hypertension who are aged over 60 years. Continued treatment of the hypertension to at least the age of 80 years has been shown to reduce the risks.[2] Thiazides are the first choice for drug treatment when dihydropyridine calcium antagonists and thiazides are contraindicated, not tolerated or ineffective.

Patients with diabetes

Studies of patients with type 2 diabetes have examined cardiovascular events as secondary events, rather than as the main endpoints. However, the comparative trials suggested that ACE inhibitors were more effective than calcium-channel antagonists in preventing cardiovascular events. As far as possible, blood pressure levels should be controlled to 140/80 mmHg or below. The Heart Outcomes Prevention Evaluation (HOPE) trial[12] found that there were significantly fewer diabetic complications (diabetic nephropathy and retinopathy) among patients with diabetes who took ramipril. The beneficial effects could not be attributed to the effects of blood pressure reduction alone, as the overall reduction was only 2–3 mmHg.

Most patients (about 80%) with diabetes would qualify for treatment with ramipril according to the conclusions of the HOPE trial. This has obvious implications for drug budgets, but could reduce the overall cost of complications of diabetes as well as providing considerable health gains.

Malignant hypertension

This is an emergency, which is fortunately rare, that has a very poor outcome if it is left untreated. Even when it is treated, a high proportion

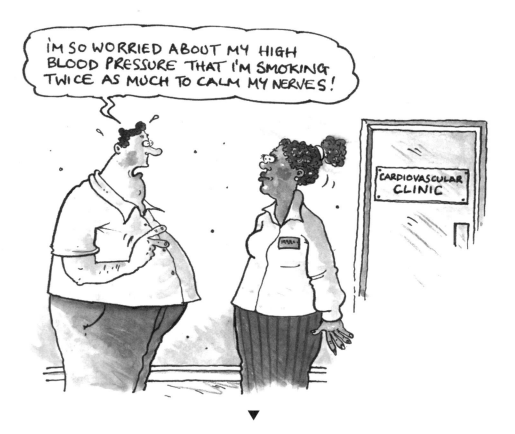

of cases go on to develop strokes or renal failure. The diagnostic criteria are a diastolic blood pressure higher than 120 mmHg, together with advanced hypertensive retinopathy (haemorrhages and exudates, with or without papilloedema). Malignant hypertension is more common in smokers and people of African-Caribbean origin. Recommended treatment includes a reduction in blood pressure over about one week to avoid precipitating a stroke by too rapid a decrease. You will probably want to seek specialist help, especially as secondary hypertension is more common in this group than in non-malignant hypertension, and patients will require investigation to exclude a precipitating cause.

Is it worth the effort?

Hypertension is an important risk factor for cardiovascular disease. In controlled trials antihypertensive drug treatment for more than 3–5 years prevents cardiovascular complications, but little is known about the long-term prognosis. A follow-up study of duration 20–22 years[13] showed that treated male patients with hypertension had significantly increased mortality, especially from coronary heart disease, compared with males without hypertension from the same population. The high incidence of coronary heart disease was related to organ damage, smoking and cholesterol levels at the time of entry to the study.

The moral is clear. Do not look at levels of blood pressure in isolation – look at the whole patient and their risk factors. Reducing blood pressure helps to prevent stroke, but other risk factors (e.g. smoking or cholesterol levels) are likely to be more important in preventing other cardiovascular adverse events.

Reflection exercises

Exercise 2

Undertake a SWOT (strengths, weaknesses, opportunities and threats) analysis of the way your practice operates its systems and procedures for managing patients with hypertension.

This will entail convening a group to represent all elements of your practice team (e.g. GP, nurse, manager/support staff, pharmacist). Then brainstorm what your strengths, weaknesses, opportunities and threats are with regard to the care of those with hypertension. You will be considering the following:

(i) your infrastructure – the practice protocol, access to and availability of nurse-led clinics, hardware and software, information resources and the capacity for computerised recall
(ii) your capability – staff numbers and posts, skills (e.g. clinical, personal, communication, IT)
(iii) your capacity – how you cope with demand (e.g. if the nurses run the hypertension clinic, who does the work that they did before?)
(iv) the extent to which you work as a team across the practice, with others from secondary care or the independent sector, and most of all with patients – including responding to feedback to achieve patient-centred care.

Use the 14 components of clinical governance described in Chapter 1 as a checklist for the SWOT analysis.

Then make a plan for improvement, including what you need to learn (and transfer your needs and action plan to your personal and practice development plans), what you need to buy, who you need to appoint or involve, and what you need to reorganise.

Exercise 3

Visit a neighbouring practice and compare how you manage hypertension in your patients with their systems and procedures.

Compare your practice protocols for the management of coronary heart disease as a whole, while you are there. Look for gaps and refine your protocols accordingly.

Exercise 4

Review the extent to which you are successful in helping patients with diabetes to gain optimal control over their blood glucose and blood pressure, and minimise complications.

Randomly select 20 case-notes from patients with type 1 diabetes, and make a further random selection of 20 case-notes from those with type 2 diabetes (controlled by oral therapy/insulin or diet) and compare how well controlled the following risk factors are compared with the goals you are aiming for:

(i) blood pressure

(ii) HbA$_{1c}$

(iii) smoking status

(iv) lipid levels (total cholesterol, HDL-cholesterol and fasting triglycerides)

(v) body mass index.

What do you and your team need to learn from this exercise, and what reorganisation of the practice do you need to make?

Now that you have completed these interactive reflection exercises, transfer the information to the empty template of the personal development plan on pages 142–151 if you are working on your own learning plan, or to the practice personal and professional development plan on pages 165–172 if you are working on a practice team learning plan. Don't forget to keep the evidence of your learning in your personal portfolio.

References

1 Fahey TP and Peters TJ (1996) What constitutes controlled hypertension? Patient based comparison of hypertension guidelines. *BMJ.* **313**: 93–6.

2 Ramsay LE, Williams B, Johnston GD *et al.* (1999) British Hypertension Society Guidelines for hypertension management 1999: summary. *BMJ.* **319**: 630–5.

3 NHS Executive (2000) *National Service Framework for Coronary Heart Disease.* Department of Health, London.

4 O'Brien E, Waeber B, Parati G *et al.* (2001) Blood pressure measuring devices: recommendations of the European Society of Hypertension. *BMJ.* **322**: 531–6.

5 Muscholl MW, Hense HW, Bröckel U *et al.* (1988) Changes in left ventricular structure and function in patients with white coat hypertension: cross sectional survey. *BMJ.* **317**: 565–70.

6 Foord-Kelcey G (ed.) (2001) *Guidelines. Volume 13.* Medenium Group Publishing Ltd., Berkhamsted.

7 Barton S (ed.) (2001) *Clinical Evidence. Issue 5.* BMJ Publishing Group, London.

8 Royal Pharmaceutical Society of Great Britain (1997) *From Compliance to Concordance: towards shared goals in medicine taking.* Royal Pharmaceutical Society of Great Britain, London.

9 Baker R (2001) Is it time to review the idea of compliance with guidelines? *Br J Gen Pract.* **51**: 7.

10 Montgomery AA, Fahey T, Peters TJ *et al.* (2000) Evaluation of computer-based clinical decision support systems and risk chart management of hypertension in primary care: randomised controlled trial. *BMJ.* **320**: 686–90.

11 Lip GYH (2000) *ABC of Hypertension* (4e). BMJ Publications, London.

12 The Heart Outcomes Prevention Evaluation (HOPE) Investigators (2000) Effects of an angiotensin-converting-enzyme inhibitor, ramipril, on cardio-vascular events in high-risk patients. *NEJM.* **342**: 1445–53.

13 Anderson OK, Almgreen T, Persoson B *et al.* (1998) Survival after treated hypertension. *BMJ.* **317**: 167–71.

CHAPTER 3

Angina

What is angina?

Angina pectoris (usually just called angina) is a recurring pain or discomfort in the chest. It feels like a pressing heavy pain or a squeezing constricting feeling, usually under the sternum, but sometimes in the neck, jaws or down the arm. People often describe the pain with a clenched fist pressed against the sternum. Attacks are often triggered by exercise or emotional stress, and occur more frequently in cold weather or after meals.

Angina is due to the heart muscle not receiving enough blood, usually because the coronary arteries are narrowed. All chest pain is not angina or a heart attack, and a useful overview of differential diagnoses is described in the *Symptom Sorter*,[1] but the doctor's nightmare is to mistakenly treat someone for presumed indigestion when in fact they have cardiac pain.

A careful history usually gives the diagnosis (*see* Table 3.1 for some help with sorting out what the underlying causes might be).

People with reflux oesophagitis usually complain of a burning pain from the lower end of the sternum upwards. Sometimes the pain is between the shoulder blades, and worse on lying down or bending over. They usually describe the pain with an open hand and the fingers travelling up the sternum.

Table 3.1 Common causes of chest pain

Cause	Worse on exercise	Worse lying down	Better after resting	Localised tenderness	Shortness of breath	Cough
Angina	Yes	No	Yes	No	Sometimes	No
Reflux oesophagitis	Sometimes	Yes	Sometimes	No	No	Sometimes
Anxiety	Variable	Variable	Variable	Sometimes	Usually	Sometimes
Musculo-skeletal	Variable	No	Worse	Marked	Sometimes	No
Pleurisy	Yes	Variable	No	No	Usual	Usual

If the angina-type pain lasts for more than a few minutes and is not relieved by resting (or the angina medication), consider whether the patient has a myocardial infarction. If the pain goes away with stretching, taking a deep breath, changing position or drinking a glass of water, it is almost certainly not angina.

After taking the history, you would normally include at least an examination of the chest, the abdomen if indicated by the history, and blood pressure recording. Pleurisy is overdiagnosed and is unlikely without another cause such as a chest infection or other serious lung condition. Common causes of chest pain include pulled muscles, anxiety spasm, and costochondritis (Tieze's syndrome). People with fractured ribs usually give a history of injury.

Other less common conditions include referred pain from peptic ulcer or biliary colic, or a viral cause such as shingles or Bornholm's disease. Rarely you may encounter serious conditions such as a pulmonary embolus, pneumothorax, cardiomyopathy, myocarditis or pericarditis, or a dissecting aneurysm.

Investigations

After a careful history and examination, the diagnosis may be quite clear. An electrocardiogram (ECG) may be completely normal at rest in angina, but may show ischaemic changes, a myocardial infarction (old or new), pericarditis or a pulmonary embolism.

If you are in doubt, then other investigations are indicated, such as a chest X-ray for chest infection, rib fracture, heart disease, cardiomyopathy or pneumothorax.

A full blood count might reveal anaemia as a possible trigger for the angina, or it might indicate another cause for the pain, such as a chest infection, pleurisy or costochondritis.

Other underlying causes of angina might be diabetes (check the blood glucose level) or hyperlipidaemia (check the serum cholesterol level).

Management of stable angina

'People with symptoms of angina or suspected angina should receive appropriate investigation and treatment to relieve their pain and reduce their risk of coronary events.'[2]

Treatment of symptoms

Immediate relief

Sublingual nitrates give immediate control of angina symptoms. Tablets are cheap but lose their efficacy on exposure to light, heat and the atmosphere, so sprays may be cost-effective if attacks of angina are infrequent.

Background therapy

The number of acute attacks can be reduced with background therapy, such as beta-blockers and/or nitrates and/or calcium antagonists.

The North of England Guidelines (described in the *Guidelines*[3] publication) suggest giving regular treatment to all except those who have only occasional attacks. The drug of first choice would be a beta-blocker, and if the patient is unable to take this because of intolerance or a contraindication such as asthma, then verapamil should be used. There is little to choose between other initial medications if neither of these is tolerated.

If symptoms are inadequately controlled, add a second drug. If the patient is on a beta-blocker, then add a calcium antagonist or, if that is not tolerated, isosorbide mononitrate. Isosorbide mononitrate can also be added to a calcium antagonist as a second-line drug. If symptoms are not controlled, refer the patient for further investigations and advice.

Reducing risk factors

The risk of progression of angina to myocardial infarction can be reduced by the following:

- stopping smoking – the use of nicotine patches seems to be safe in people with coronary heart disease[4]
- lifestyle changes, such as increasing physical exercise,[5] diet and weight control
- controlling blood pressure (*see* Chapter 2)
- low-dose aspirin (75 mg daily)
- reducing serum cholesterol levels to below 5 mmol/L (especially keeping the low-density lipoprotein C concentration below 3 mmol/L) or reducing the level by 30% (whichever is greater).

Patients need information about the symptoms of a heart attack (*see* Chapter 4) and how it differs from their angina attacks, so that in the event of a heart attack they can seek help rapidly via the 999 emergency telephone system.

Driving

Patients who have no angina at rest or at the wheel of a car do not need to stop driving socially. Those patients whose employment is dependent on their public service vehicle (PSV) or heavy goods vehicle (HGV) licence will need early referral for exercise testing, and will need to notify the Driver and Vehicle Licensing Agency.[6] They may need help with alternative employment either from their employer or from the disability employment service at the employment offices of the Department of Social Security. The regulations include the following advice.

- If drug treatment for any cardiovascular condition is required, then any adverse effect which may affect driver performance will disqualify them.
- An applicant or driver who has, after cardiac assessment, been permitted to hold either an LGV or a PCV licence will usually be issued with a short-term licence (maximum duration 3 years) that is renewable on receipt of satisfactory medical reports.
- Exercise evaluation must be performed on a bicycle or treadmill. Drivers should be able to complete three stages of the Bruce protocol or equivalent safely, without anti-anginal medication for 48 hours, and should remain free from signs of cardiovascular dysfunction (i.e. angina pectoris, syncope, hypotension, sustained ventricular tachycardia and/or electrocardiographic ST-segment shift, which accredited medical opinion interprets as being indicative of myocardial ischaemia).
- In the presence of established coronary heart disease, exercise evaluation will be required at regular intervals not to exceed 3 years.
- If the cause of the chest pain is in doubt, an exercise test should be performed as described above. Patients with a locomotor disorder who cannot comply will require specialist cardiological opinion
- Angiography is not required for (re-)licensing purposes in patients with coronary heart disease.

Referral for further investigations and treatment

Many areas now have 'rapid-access' clinics for the evaluation of chest pain.

Box 3.1

Bandolier (*see* Appendix 3 for a list of useful websites) gives an account of a rapid-access chest pain clinic which was set up because waiting times for cardiology clinics were putting patients at risk.[7] Discussion between local GPs and the department of cardiology led to a clinic being set up to see patients with the diagnosis of possible stable angina. The clinic was open every day between 12 noon and 2 p.m. to see men over the age of 30 years and women over the age of 40 years with recent-onset chest pain (within the last 2–4 weeks) and no previous history of treatment for coronary heart disease. Patients' details were faxed from primary care to the clinic, and patients were seen within 24 hours. The diagnostic tests were all performed at that attendance, and a computer-based pro forma was completed. This generated a semi-structured report that was faxed back to the GP as soon as the consultation was completed. The fax included the diagnosis made, the risk factors, investigation results and recommended treatment. Where hospital-based care and treatment were needed, this was arranged for the regular cardiology clinic. The service was well regarded by both patients and GPs, with 80% of GPs preferring this arrangement. In total, 69% of patients seen had chest pain of non-cardiac origin. Few patients required further hospital investigations or treatment, but the clinic had little impact on the workload of the regular cardiology clinics.

Useful guidelines and flow charts for the investigation of a patient with suspected angina appear in the publication, *Guidelines*,[3] or in the Scottish Intercollegiate Guidelines Network (SIGN) guidelines (*Guidelines No. 32*[8]) (*see* list of useful websites in Appendix 3). PRODIGY gives extensive and detailed guidelines for those with access to them via their surgery computer system or on a website (*see* Appendix 3). You may want to adapt these together with others in your primary care organisation for local use, taking into account the availability of an open-access clinic or cardiological out-patient facilities, and demand better access and provision if necessary.

Medical treatment is effective for most people with angina, and is the only option for those who are frail or otherwise unsuitable for revascularisation. Referral for an exercise test can help to differentiate those with more severe disease. Those with major abnormalities on an exercise test would then go on to have carotid angiography. Refer for angiography those patients with angina that persists despite optimal medical treatment and lifestyle advice. The results of arteriography determine whether angioplasty or bypass grafting will be beneficial. *Clinical Evidence*[4] discusses the benefits and risks of these procedures, but in practice the specialist service will make the decision as to whether to offer it. However, you need to be able to discuss the relevance of the evidence with individual patients.

Box 3.2

There is good evidence that percutaneous transluminal coronary angioplasty (PTCA) improves the symptoms of angina, but there is no evidence that it reduces the overall incidence of death or myocardial infarction in people with stable angina.[4] Coronary artery bypass grafting (CABG) was associated with greater risks of death in the first year, but reduced the risk of death at 5 and 10 years. As most of the studies were performed on selected groups under 65 years of age, it is difficult to know to what extent the results can be generalised to older people. Intracoronary stents have more recently shown better results than PTCA, since the control of thrombosis and bleeding complications has been improved.

Very extensive distal coronary artery disease or very poor ventricular function may preclude attempts at revascularisation.

The *Effective Health Care Bulletin* on the management of stable angina[9] commented that there was evidence of unequal access to testing and revascularisation with regard to gender, ethnic group and social class. Promoting equity requires the systematic documentation of the process of investigation and treatment to ensure equal access. Although men have a higher incidence of angina than do women, and develop it at a younger age, it is important not to forget the risks in women, particularly after the menopause. Exercise tests seem to be less reliable in women, for reasons that are not yet understood. People of South Asian descent living in the UK have a higher risk of angina (about 40%) and those of African-Caribbean descent have a lower risk (estimated to be 25–50%) than Caucasian members of the UK in general. People of higher social class do not have higher risks of angina (although those in sedentary occupations may do), but are more frequently referred for testing and revascularisation.

You should have a particularly low threshold of suspicion for angina in people with diabetes, so enquire pro-actively for symptoms at their routine check-ups. Diabetics have a fivefold increased risk of dying from coronary heart disease compared with individuals of their sex and age without diabetes.

Unstable angina

Angina may appear as a severe first episode or as frequently recurring bouts of pain. The previous pattern of stable angina may change in that episodes become more severe, last longer, are provoked by less exercise or start occurring at rest. This is sometimes called crescendo angina or pre-infarction angina. Patients need to know that these symptoms may signal a significant increase in their risk of having a myocardial infarction. Referral to a cardiologist or rapid-access clinic is usually indicated.

There is a review of treatments for unstable angina in *Clinical Evidence*.[4] As well as the treatments advised for stable angina (e.g. low-dose aspirin), ticlopidine was found to be more effective than conventional treatment without aspirin, but was associated with a significant risk of provoking neutropenia. Ticlopidine may be an alternative treatment for individuals who are intolerant of or allergic to aspirin, but must be initiated by a specialist. Other treatments will also be provided by secondary care services (e.g. low-molecular-weight heparin, hirudin, revascularisation or glycoprotein inhibitors). There is no evidence that calcium-channel blockers prevent death or myocardial infarction in patients with unstable angina.

Variant angina (Prinzmetal's angina)

Unlike typical angina, attacks are usually very painful and occur at rest, generally between midnight and breakfast-time. Variant angina is strongly associated with the development of myocardial infarction, cardiac arrhythmias and death. It is due to spasm of the coronary arteries, and two-thirds of patients with variant angina have severe atherosclerosis of at least one coronary vessel. The sufferers usually go through an active period of severe symptoms for about 6 months or so. During this time they are at high risk of a non-fatal myocardial infarction (20% of cases) or death (up to 10% of cases), especially if a serious arrhythmia develops.

Most people who survive this acute phase settle down into a stable pattern with few symptoms. Long-term survival is good after this acute phase, especially if the coronary arteries are not significantly affected by atherosclerosis.

Investigation and treatment should be as advised for unstable angina.

Reflection exercises

Exercise 5

Having read through the material in this chapter, do you have a good understanding about how to manage an individual patient with angina and when to refer them? Or do you need to read and study more?

You could look up the original references cited here.

Exercise 6

Find out what initiatives have been undertaken by any of the practice team to ascertain patients' views in the previous 12 months.

This might have included surveying or involving anyone registered with the practice (regular patients, people who do not use the services, carers) or the local community. How was the information gained from the initiative used? Did changes result? Your own or practice team members' learning needs from this exercise might include the following:

(i) learning more about the variety of methods that can be employed to find out patients' views

(ii) learning how to apply any of those methods to find out the views of people with angina about the care or services provided or that they wish to receive

(iii) learning more about using a survey so that the findings are useful in making changes to the way services are planned or delivered, or staff behave (e.g. when a patient presents complaining of chest pain)

(iv) learning more about involving individual patients in decision making about the management of their angina.

Use these learning exercises to gather the views of people suffering from angina about one or more aspects of the way in which you provide care or services. Discuss the information you have obtained with the practice team, and plan how to make improvements in your services.

Now that you have completed these interactive reflection exercises, transfer the information to the relevant section about your learning needs in the empty template on pages 142–151 if you are working on your own personal development plan, or to the practice personal and professional development plan on pages 165–172 if you are working on a practice team learning plan. Don't forget to keep the evidence of your learning in your personal portfolio.

References

1 Hopcroft K and Forte V (1999) *Symptom Sorter.* Radcliffe Medical Press, Oxford.

2 NHS Executive (2000) *National Service Framework for Coronary Heart Disease.* Department of Health, London.

3 Foord-Kelcey G (ed.) (2001) *Guidelines. Volume 13.* Medenium Group Publishing Ltd., Berkhamsted.

4 Barton S (ed.) (2001) *Clinical Evidence. Issue 5.* BMJ Publishing Group, London.

5 Jolliffe JA, Rees K, Taylor RS *et al.* (2001) Exercise rehabilitation for coronary heart disease. In: *The Cochrane Library.* Update Software, Oxford.

6 Drivers Medical Unit DVLA (1999) *At a Glance Guide to Current Medical Standards of Fitness to Drive.* Driver and Vehicle Licensing Agency, Swansea.

7 Jain D, Fluck D, Sayer JW *et al.* (1997) One-stop chest pain clinic can identify high cardiac risk. *J R Coll Physicians Lond.* **31**: 401–4.

8 Scottish Intercollegiate Guidelines Network (1998) *Coronary Revascularisation in the Management of Stable Angina Pectoralis. Guidelines No 32.* Scottish Intercollegiate Guidelines Network, Edinburgh.

9 NHS Centre for Reviews and Dissemination (1997) Management of stable angina. In: *Effective Health Care Bulletin.* University of York, York.

CHAPTER 4

Myocardial infarction

What is acute myocardial infarction?

Acute myocardial infarction (AMI) is the sudden occlusion of a coronary artery, leading to myocardial death.[1] An atheromatous plaque may become unstable causing thrombosis and occlusion. It causes severe chest pain, that persists at rest and despite nitrates. Nausea and vomiting are common. Pain may radiate into the jaw, back, upper abdomen, or one or both arms.[2,3]

The signs of a myocardial infarction are those of an autonomic disturbance, namely pallor, sweating, breathlessness and tachycardia. There may be extrasystoles or a third heart sound, syncope or cardiac arrest. It is extremely difficult to make an accurate diagnosis when chest pain presents. Not all prolonged chest pain is due to ischaemia, and not all angina attacks lead to infarction, as the study described in Box 4.1 illustrates. Chapter 3 gives more information about the differential diagnosis of chest pain.

Sometimes people have no chest pain, in which case their infarction is described as 'silent'. This is more common in elderly people and those with diabetes.

Box 4.1 Not all protracted chest pain is a myocardial infarction[4]

One study of patients seen at an Accident and Emergency department illustrates the wide spectrum of types of chest pain that present as 'emergencies'. Half of the patients presenting with 'chest pain', 'angina' or 'heart attack' were admitted. Of these, one-fifth had had an acute myocardial infarction, one-third had angina and the rest had a non-cardiac cause accounting for their pain.

Ischaemic heart disease (IHD) is the commonest cause of death worldwide. It accounts for over 20% of all deaths in the UK. About one-third of those who have an acute myocardial infarction die from it. Around 20% die before seeking or receiving medical attention, and about 10–15% die in hospital. Most in-hospital deaths occur during the first 2 days after admission. Around 70% of all coronary heart disease deaths occur outside hospital.[1,5]

The cause of death is usually ventricular arrhythmias, myocardial rupture or cardiac pump failure. Other complications include congestive heart failure, cardiogenic shock, non-fatal arrhythmias and valvular dysfunction.[1]

Investigations

The diagnosis of acute myocardial infarction can usually be made on the basis of the presenting symptoms and signs. Chest pain is generally more severe and prolonged than for angina.

Immediate investigations

ECG

The electrocardiogram (ECG) can confirm the myocardial infarction by characteristic changes. However, a normal ECG does not exclude an evolving myocardial infarction. Elevation of the ST-segment over the area of the infarct usually (but not always) occurs during the first hour of chest pain, or the onset of bundle-branch block. A Q-wave usually develops during the subsequent 24 hours and persists indefinitely. The ST-segment usually returns to normal within a few days of the attack, and T-wave inversion may occur. Changes in other leads pinpoint the location of the coronary artery with the occlusion. Serial ECGs can be used to monitor the extension of the infarction as well as recovery.[6]

If a coronary artery is only partially blocked, there may be ST-segment depression or T-wave inversion on the ECG.

Cardiac enzymes

Cardiac enzymes are released from the infarcted myocardium. Creatinine phosphokinase (CPK), cardiac troponins T and I (highly specific and sensitive markers of myocardial necrosis) and glutamic oxaloacetic transaminase (GOT) levels tend to peak at 24 hours after infarction, and levels fall over the subsequent 3 to 6 days. Levels of CPK can be raised when skeletal muscle is damaged (e.g. in patients receiving intra-muscular injections (so give analgesia intravenously rather than by the intramuscular route). Liver, kidney, brain or lung disease can increase GOT levels and lead to a misdiagnosis of myocardial infarction if GOT levels are used in isolation.

Longer-term investigations

Coronary angiography

High-risk patients should be considered for coronary angiography as a preliminary to revascularisation. This patient group includes those who have angina or significant changes in an exercise ECG or isotope perfusion imaging after a myocardial infarction.

Exercise testing

An exercise test will identify reversible ischaemia, even if the patient does not experience angina. Routine exercise testing at the time of hospital discharge helps to identify which patients are at risk of complications, and who will benefit from early angiography and coronary artery bypass grafting or angioplasty.

Treatment

Immediate treatment for acute myocardial infarction

The priorities of treatment for a patient with suspected myocardial infarction are to ensure rapid access to a defibrillator in case they suffer a cardiac arrest, and to relieve their chest pain and their anxiety.

Lives can be saved if a patient arrests in the presence of a person with a defibrillator. The siting of defibrillators in public places such as railway stations and shopping centres is being considered, as modern defibrillators can be used by lay people with minimal training.[7]

Although there is a national trend towards the increasing use of 999 calls for chest pain, there is often considerable delay and public misunderstanding about the urgency of obtaining expert help for prolonged chest pain. Even if there is a small risk of a myocardial infarction, the emergency ambulance should be called with a clear message that the patient should be targeted for an 8-minutes response. An 'urgent request' is of lower priority than the 8-minutes response request, and 999 calls are all treated as emergencies. Therefore we should all be taking every opportunity to educate the general public, especially those with known heart disease, to encourage them to seek medical assistance for chest pain as early as possible.

Patients with suspected acute myocardial infarction should receive the following:

- pain relief with an intravenous opiate (e.g. intravenous diamorphine 2.5 to 5.0 mg) and an anti-emetic (e.g. metoclopramide 10 mg); in the absence of a GP, most ambulance services are authorised to use nalbuphine
- aspirin (300 mg orally) chewed before swallowing
- oxygen
- plenty of reassurance to relieve their anxiety and distress.

Studies estimate that one life is saved for every 40 people treated with aspirin during the acute phase of the infarction.[1]

Pre-hospital thrombolysis with anistreplase or urokinase is being piloted but is not generally available. This may have more of a place in rural areas, where there will be more than a 30-minute delay in getting the patient to hospital.

Immediate post-myocardial infarction treatment

Thrombolytic treatment

Thrombolytic drugs activate the conversion of plasminogen to plasmin, which degrades fibrin and breaks down clots.

Patients who survive an acute myocardial infarction (MI) should be given thrombolysis, provided that the ECG meets specified criteria indicating that an MI has occurred. Prompt thrombolytic treatment with a drug (e.g. streptokinase, alteplase or reteplase) within 6 hours, and perhaps up to 12 hours or longer, after the onset of symptoms can restore blood flow through a previously occluded artery, thus reducing mortality from acute myocardial infarction. A total of 56 people would need to be treated with thrombolytic drugs in the acute phase of myocardial infarction in order to prevent one additional death.[1]

The choice of thrombolytic drug is generally determined by the local protocol. The adverse effects of thrombolytic treatment in the acute phase are such that there is one additional stroke for every 250 people treated and one additional major bleed for every 143 people treated. Intracranial haemorrhage is more common in older people, those with low body weight and those suffering from hypertension on admission to hospital.[1]

Contraindications to thrombolysis include previous haemorrhagic stroke, any stroke within the previous 6 months, arterial or other surgery within 1 month, active peptic ulcer or other internal bleeding, oesophageal varices and pregnancy.[2,3]

Beta-blocker drugs

All patients with acute myocardial infarction should be started on a beta-blocker drug immediately and continued indefinitely, unless there is a contraindication (e.g. asthma). Beta-blockers protect against sudden death in patients who have any degree of risk of ischaemic heart disease after a myocardial infarction. Treatment with beta-blockers within hours of acute myocardial infarction reduces both the mortality and reinfarction rates, by reducing rates of cardiac rupture and ventricular fibrillation.[1] Adding beta-blockers to thrombolytic treatment may confer additional benefits. There are long-term benefits in the prevention of the order of 12 deaths for every 1000 patients treated in the first year.

Emergency revascularisation

If chest pain persists after a myocardial infarction, despite treatment, refer the patient for arteriography to determine whether the coronary arteries are blocked or narrowed. Alternatives that may be considered are percutaneous transluminal coronary angioplasty (PTCA) to reopen a narrowed coronary artery, or coronary artery bypass grafting (CABG) of one or more coronary arteries. Vascular disease may also require valve replacement.

There is some evidence that primary PTCA is at least as effective as thrombolysis in the treatment of acute myocardial infarction, in terms of reducing rates of mortality, reinfarction and stroke. However, the research evidence was derived from studies conducted in specialist centres, and the favourable outcomes from PTCA may not be reproducible in non-specialist PTCA treatment centres.[1] The implanting of coronary stents at the time of primary angioplasty further improves clinical outcome, as coronary angioplasty and bypass grafting are less likely to be needed in the future.

Longer-term post-myocardial infarction treatment

Agree or review the practice's or primary care organisation's secondary prevention protocol for patients who have sustained a myocardial infarction to ensure that:

- secondary prevention is instituted in a systematic way
- drug treatment (e.g. choice of statins and threshold for treatment) is consistent
- recording of information systems and definitions are consistent within the primary care team and hopefully across the primary care organisation and secondary care sector
- patients receive consistent advice
- patients are followed up and encouraged to adhere to the treatment regimes for which there is most evidence
- the blood pressure and blood sugar levels of patients with diabetes are meticulously controlled
- all patients are offered a programme of cardiac rehabilitation. The programme should start in hospital and be provided by specialist multidisciplinary staff. It should be clear which aspects of post-infarction care the hospital is responsible for, and which aspects those working in primary care have agreed to take on.[2,7,8]

(*See* Chapter 8 for more information about secondary prevention).

Medication unless contraindicated

Starting ACE inhibitors promptly (e.g. within 24 hours) after myocardial infarction reduces death rates in both the short and longer terms. These effects persist even if ACE inhibitors are discontinued after a few weeks.

Unless there are contraindications, all patients should take an ACE inhibitor indefinitely following a myocardial infarction. The evidence is most robust for the following:

- ACE inhibitors taken for around 6 weeks following myocardial infarction
- indefinite use of these drugs by patients who have left ventricular dysfunction.

Aspirin should be taken indefinitely if myocardial infarction or other atherosclerotic disease is confirmed. Consider clopidogrel if aspirin is contraindicated.[9]

A statin should be started before discharge from hospital if the patient has a cholesterol level of 5.0 mmol/L or higher.[8,10]

Calcium-channel blockers have not been shown to increase survival or outcome.[1]

Box 4.2 A district-wide audit of the management of patients after myocardial infarction (MI)[11]

A total of 311 patients were included in the audit. Criteria were based on the Standing Medical Advisory Committee (SMAC) guidelines on the use of statins,[12] and the *British National Formulary*.[13] In total, 76% of general practices in North Staffordshire agreed to be visited by the project facilitator who collected the data.

- 86% of patients had at least one serum cholesterol result recorded in their patient record post-MI.
- 62% of patients had a total cholesterol result recorded that had been measured within 3 months of their MI.
- 60% of patients had started on a statin after MI, or were already taking a statin prior to their MI.
- 50% of 195 patients who had had a total cholesterol result recorded within 3 months of their MI had a measurement below 4.8 mmol/L.
- 95% of patients had had at least one blood pressure measurement recorded since their MI. For 45% of patients, their last blood pressure measurement was below 140/85 mmHg.
- 95% of patients had a record of being treated with aspirin at the time of or after discharge.
- 74% of patients had a record of being treated with a beta-blocker at the time of or after discharge.
- 77% of patients had a record of smoking status post-MI.
- 28% of patients whose smoking status was recorded were still smoking.

(Data on ACE inhibitors were not collected)

Cardiac rehabilitation

Cardiac rehabilitation can reduce the risk of death by around 20–25% over subsequent years. It includes psychological support, verbal and written information about coronary heart disease, detailed advice and help tailored to the individual patient with regard to cigarette smoking, weight loss, diet and exercise. The cardiac rehabilitation programme should start in hospital under the management of a specialist, multi-disciplinary team and continue in primary care. It should be offered to the patient's partner and family as well.[6]

Reflection exercises

Exercise 7

Are all the members of the practice team (including the receptionists and other non-clinical staff) familiar with your practice protocol for dealing with someone who has a suspected myocardial infarction?

If not, review your guidelines or protocol at a practice team meeting. Ensure that everyone knows what their roles and responsibilities are.

Undertake an audit of five patients who have had a myocardial infarction in the last 12 months. Look back at their medical notes to see how long it took for them to be admitted to hospital from the time of the onset of their symptoms. Also determine whether they have been monitored and managed post-myocardial infarction according to your practice protocol.

Exercise 8

Undertake an audit of 20 people on your coronary heart disease register who are classified as having had a myocardial infarction at least one year ago.

Compare how you monitor the care of your patients post-myocardial infarction with the recommendations in the evidence-based review criteria for the primary care management of coronary heart disease in a clinical practice evaluation programme produced by the Royal College of General Practitioners.[14] For how many of your patients do you have records for the criteria listed below? For how many are you achieving excellent control or care?

Clinical assessment

* The percentage of patients post-myocardial infarction who have had their serum lipids measured.

- The percentage of patients post-myocardial infarction whose blood pressure is maintained below 140/85 mmHg where appropriate.
- The percentage of patients post-myocardial infarction who have had their blood glucose levels measured.

Therapy

- The percentage of patients post-myocardial infarction who have been treated with aspirin 75 mg daily, unless contraindicated.
- The percentage of patients post-myocardial infarction who have been treated with a beta-blocker, unless contraindicated.
- The percentage of patients post-myocardial infarction with symptomatic heart failure and evidence of impaired left ventricular function who have been treated with an ACE inhibitor, unless contraindicated.
- For those whose total cholesterol level remains > 5 mmol/L and/or LDL cholesterol > 3 mmol/L, even after dietary advice for at least 6 weeks – the percentage of patients post-myocardial infarction who have been considered for treatment with a statin, unless contraindicated.

Advice

- The percentage of patients post-myocardial infarction who smoke and have been advised to stop.
- The percentage of patients post-myocardial infarction who have been advised to take moderate exercise within their capabilities, to improve their general fitness and well-being.

Now that you have completed these interactive reflection exercises, transfer the information to the empty template of the personal development plan on pages 142–151 if you are working on your own learning plan, or to the practice personal and professional development plan on pages 165–172 if you are working on a practice team learning plan. Don't forget to keep the evidence of your learning in your personal portfolio.

References

1 Barton S (ed.) (2001) *Clinical Evidence. Issue 5.* BMJ Publishing Group, London.

2 British Cardiac Society and Royal College of Physicians (1994) The management of acute myocardial infarction: guidelines and audit standards. *J R Coll Physicians Lond.* **28**: 312–7.

3 Foord-Kelcey G (ed.) (2001) *Guidelines. Volume 13.* Medenium Group Publishing Ltd, Berkhamsted.

4 Norris RM (2000) The GP's role in acute myocardial infarction. *Practitioner.* **244**: 510–37.

5 Coats A and Chua TP (1998) *Managing the Post-Myocardial Infarct Patient.* Science Press, London.

6 Collier J (2000) Tackling myocardial infarction. *Drug Ther Bull.* **38**: 17–22.

7 NHS Executive (2000) *National Service Framework for Coronary Heart Disease.* Department of Health, London.

8 Iqbal Z, Chambers R and Woodmansey P (2001) *Implementing the National Service Framework for Coronary Heart Disease in Primary Care.* Radcliffe Medical Press, Oxford.

9 CAPRIE Steering Committee (1996) A randomised, blinded, trial of clopidogrel versus aspirin in patients at risk of ischaemic events (CAPRIE). *Lancet.* **348**: 1329–39.

10 Wood D, Durrington P, Poulter N *et al.* (1998) Joint British recommendations on prevention of coronary heart disease in clinical practice. *Heart.* **80 (Supplement 2)**: S1–29.

11 North Staffordshire Medical Audit Advisory Group (2000) *Management of Patients Post-Myocardial Infarction.* North Staffordshire Medical Audit Advisory Group, Stoke-on-Trent.

12 Standing Medical Advisory Committee (1997) *The Use of Statins.* Department of Health, Leeds.

13 Mehta D (ed.) (2001) *British National Formulary.* British Medical Association and the Royal Pharmaceutical Society of Great Britain, London.

14 Royal College of General Practitioners (2000) *Evidence-Based Review Criteria for the Primary Care Management of Coronary Heart Disease. Clinical practice evaluation programme.* Royal College of General Practitioners, London.

CHAPTER 5

Heart failure

What is heart failure?

Heart failure is a common and deadly disease. It occurs when the heart no longer maintains cardiac output or pumps blood around the body at a sufficient rate to meet metabolic requirements.

Heart failure occurs for the first time in up to 0.4% of the adult population per year. It is commoner in older age groups because improvements in the management of myocardial infarction mean that more people survive and develop heart failure. The prevalence of heart failure among those over 65 years of age living in the UK is 40 per 1000 men and 30 per 1000 women. In those aged over 80 years the prevalence is 100 per 1000 individuals. Left ventricular systolic dysfunction without symptoms occurs in 3% of the general population.[1,2]

The symptoms of heart failure are breathlessness that is worse on lying down and on exertion, ankle swelling, and cough with copious white sputum and fatigue. The most specific signs of heart failure are an elevated jugular venous pressure and a displaced apex beat. Other clinical signs, which can be found in other conditions as well, are crackles at the lung bases, peripheral oedema and third or fourth heart sounds. Misdiagnosis is common, due to either missing the diagnosis of heart failure or labelling other conditions as heart failure. Box 5.1 shows a simple version of an international classification of heart failure symptoms.

Box 5.1 Simplified version of the New York Heart Association classification of heart failure symptoms[3]

Class I
No limitations – ordinary physical activity does not cause symptoms.

Class II
Slight limitation of physical activity.

> *Class III*
> Marked limitation of physical activity.
>
> *Class IV*
> Inability to engage in any physical activity without discomfort.

Causes of heart failure

Heart failure is caused by systolic or diastolic dysfunction.

The commonest cause of heart failure is coronary artery disease. Other causes include the following:

- hypertension
- valvular disease
- cor pulmonale
- cardiomyopathy (including idiopathic)
- drugs and alcohol.

Left ventricular hypertrophy, cigarette smoking, hyperlipidaemia and diabetes mellitus are all risk factors for heart failure.

Conditions which mimic heart failure include non-cardiac causes such as the following:

- drug-induced water retention (e.g. from non-steroidal anti-inflammatory drugs and calcium-channel blockers)
- physiological oedema in women
- renal disease
- liver disease
- pulmonary disease
- anaemia
- thyroid disease
- obesity
- bilateral renal artery stenosis.

Prognosis

The prognosis of heart failure is poor. Heart failure is the single commonest cause of hospital admission in the UK. It accounts for 5% of all adult medical admissions to hospital in the UK; one-sixth of patients are readmitted with heart failure within 6 months of their first admission. Around 26–75% of patients with heart failure will have died within 5 years of its onset, according to different research studies. Ventricular arrhythmias may trigger sudden death.[1,2]

Investigations[1–4]

The National Service Framework for coronary heart disease for England states that all patients with heart failure should receive a 'full package of appropriate investigation and treatment'. Those with suspected heart failure should be offered electrocardiography or echocardiography to confirm or refute the diagnosis.

You will need to investigate any patient with suspected heart failure in order to:

- confirm or exclude the diagnosis of heart failure
- define the precise underlying cause of heart failure if possible
- identify factors which alleviate or worsen the condition
- aid management and treatment decisions
- provide baseline information for future monitoring
- obtain prognostic information.

A diagnosis of heart failure is unlikely if there is nothing in the history or examination to suggest that there is anything wrong with the heart. Many such patients are mistakenly categorised as having heart failure. It is most important to identify a cause for the heart failure.

If a patient was well before they suffered a myocardial infarction, and afterwards they appear to have developed heart failure clinically, then the clinical diagnosis is obvious and no sophisticated tests are required.

Routine blood investigations

These include the following:

- full blood count
- biochemical profile (urine and electrolytes, plasma/serum creatinine, liver enzymes, cholesterol and blood glucose levels)
- thyroid function tests.

Weight

A rapid increase in body weight may indicate worsening heart failure, whilst weight loss may suggest over-diuresis.

Chest X-ray

A chest X-ray will show cardiac enlargement, pulmonary venous congestion or pulmonary oedema. However, chest X-rays have a limited value in the diagnosis of heart failure. Cardiomegaly signifies the presence of heart disease but does not identify the cause of heart failure. Significant left ventricular dysfunction may occur in the absence of cardiomegaly.

ECG

Left ventricular dysfunction is very rare in the presence of a normal 12-lead ECG. However, an abnormal ECG does not mean that the patient has heart failure.

Echocardiography[5]

Echocardiography involves taking a moving picture of the heart by reflected ultrasound. These pictures require expert interpretation. Echocardiography provides an accurate assessment of left ventricular systolic dysfunction, and may also demonstrate features of diastolic dysfunction.

Echocardiography can be used to:

- establish the cause of heart failure in a patient when the diagnosis is in doubt
- show whether there are structural abnormalities of the heart which might be responsible for heart failure, so providing circumstantial evidence that a patient's symptoms are due to heart failure
- aid the investigation of breathlessness
- assess the significance of heart murmurs
- screen healthy people who have a family history of cardiomyopathy.

Box 5.2

The majority of patients who are diagnosed with heart failure currently do not have echocardiography to determine whether they have left ventricular systolic dysfunction. In a study of 600 patients who were labelled as having heart failure, only 25% had definite left ventricular dysfunction. In total, 23 of the patients who were labelled as having heart failure had atrial fibrillation, and most (60%) of those had normal left ventricular function. A further 20% had valvular abnormalities.[6]

Radionuclide ventriculography[5]

Isotope or radionuclide studies represent the most accurate and reproducible technique for assessment of left ventricular systolic dysfunction. They can be used to investigate left ventricular function, as they provide slightly more information than echocardiography. Because of the expense and the time taken, radionuclide ventriculography is not routinely indicated in the investigation of suspected heart failure.

Radionuclide investigations are more commonly used to look for exercise-induced ischaemia in cases where the ECG is unhelpful.

Treatment of heart failure[1–4,7,8]

The National Service Framework for coronary heart disease for England recommends that all patients with confirmed heart failure should receive treatments that are likely to relieve symptoms and reduce their risk of death.

Angiotensin-converting-enzyme (ACE) inhibitors

All patients with symptoms of heart failure and/or evidence of impaired left ventricular function should be treated with an ACE inhibitor. These drugs are associated with a 24% reduction in death rates in patients with heart failure.

There is no evidence of any clinically important differences or benefits between different ACE inhibitor drugs, so patients should be treated with the cheapest ACE inhibitor that they can tolerate at the recommended therapeutic doses. The relative beneficial effects of ACE inhibitors are also similar in different subgroups of people.

ACE inhibitors can delay the development of symptomatic heart failure and reduce cardiovascular events in patients with asymptomatic left ventricular systolic dysfunction, and in those with other cardiovascular risk factors.

The main adverse effects of ACE inhibitors are cough, hypotension, hyperkalaemia and renal dysfunction.

Angiotensin-II-receptor antagonists

None of these types of drugs are licensed in the UK for use in heart failure. It is not clear whether they should be used instead of or in addition to an ACE inhibitor.

The evidence supports the use of angiotensin-II-receptor blockers in patients who cannot tolerate ACE inhibitors. We know that this should improve their heart failure symptoms, but we do not know whether it reduces death rates, and research into this is still ongoing.

Box 5.3 Clinical effectiveness in the real world[9]

A total of 21 GPs in one locality worked together to review their management of patients with heart failure. National guidelines were individualised for local use after discussions with all local GPs, echocardiography technicians, cardiologists and pharmacists. A baseline survey of GPs' views, as well as audit of management against the guidelines, revealed inconsistencies between the way in which GPs believed that heart failure should be managed and the way in which they actually managed it. Most GPs were familiar with the evidence for prescribing ACE inhibitors, yet fewer than 50% were prescribing these drugs routinely to diagnosed patients. In the re-audit 1 year later, more diagnosed patients were receiving echocardiograms, although there was no change in the proportion of patients who were considered for ACE inhibitors.

Diuretics

Patients with signs of sodium and water retention (e.g. peripheral oedema) should receive diuretic therapy.

Combining ACE inhibitors and diuretics results in:

- improved signs and symptoms of all grades of heart failure
- improved exercise tolerance
- slowing down of the progression from mild to severe heart failure
- reduced hospital admission rates
- improved survival in all grades of heart failure
- better cardiac function.

Low-dose (25 mg) spironolactone should be considered in patients who are already being treated with diuretics, an ACE inhibitor and/or digoxin, or who have moderate or severe heart failure (New York Heart Association classifications III and IV; *see* Box 5.1). Adding spironolactone has been shown to decrease mortality and reduce the rate of hospital admissions.

Beta-blocker drugs[10,11]

Beta-blocker drugs are licensed for use in heart failure. They should be considered in patients who are already being treated with diuretics and/or digoxin and an ACE inhibitor, and who are clinically stable and in mild to moderate failure (New York Heart Association classification I to III; *see* Box 5.1). Beta-blocker drugs need to be started at a low dose that is titrated up over a period of weeks or months. Patients should be closely supervised (e.g. by fortnightly examination and review), as beta-blockers can worsen heart failure. If specialist supervision is impracticable in view of the large numbers of patients involved, local shared-care protocols should be developed by cardiac specialists and those in primary care.

Adding beta-blocker drugs to standard treatment with ACE inhibitors in patients with moderate heart failure reduces the risk of death and hospital admissions.

At present, bisoprolol and carvedilol are licensed for use in heart failure. Metoprolol has been used in research studies, but is *not* licensed for use in the treatment of heart failure in the UK.

It will take much education and experience before the majority of general practitioners are comfortable about prescribing beta-blocker drugs for patients with heart failure, as this prescribing approach is contrary to that which they learned about and practised as students and younger doctors. The workload implications for GPs of personally supervising beta-blocker prescribing to patients with chronic heart failure are huge, and may be insurmountable for many general practice teams.

Digoxin

Digoxin decreases the rate of hospital admissions for worsening heart failure in patients who are already receiving diuretics and ACE inhibitors. There is no evidence that digoxin affects mortality.

Digoxin is used for:

- all patients with heart failure and atrial fibrillation who need to have their ventricular rate controlled, and who cannot take beta-blockers
- patients with moderately severe or severely symptomatic heart failure who remain symptomatic despite diuretic and ACE inhibitor therapy, who have had more than one hospital admission for heart failure, or who have very poor left ventricular systolic function or persisting cardiomegaly
- patients with heart failure who have been treated with a diuretic but are unable to tolerate an ACE inhibitor or an angiotensin-II-receptor antagonist.

Patients who have already been treated with a diuretic and/or digoxin, but who are truly intolerant of an ACE inhibitor and angiotensin II, should be considered for hydralazine and isosorbide dinitrate combination therapy.

Calcium-channel blocker drugs

These drugs do not appear to be of any benefit for patients with heart failure, and they should be avoided. They appear to exacerbate symptoms of heart failure or increase mortality in patients with pulmonary congestion after myocardial infarction.

Anti-arrhythmic treatment

There is some inconclusive evidence that amiodarone reduces total mortality in patients with heart failure. Other anti-arrhythmic drugs may increase mortality in patients with heart failure.

Revascularisation/transplantation

Subgroups of heart failure patients may benefit from revascularisation/surgical transplantation.

General lifestyle advice for patients with heart failure

1 Avoid salt-rich foods.
2 Try regular exercise that is specifically tailored for people with heart failure if there are no contraindications.
3 Alcohol is contraindicated in alcohol-induced cardiomyopathy, but otherwise it may be taken in small quantities (1–2 units per day).
4 Stop smoking.
5 Aim for small stepwise changes towards modest weight loss targets if obese.

Box 5.4 Improving the management of heart failure[12]

A multidisciplinary initiative in North Derbyshire improved the management of heart failure as measured by prescribing data for ACE inhibitors and diuretics, referrals for echocardiography, admissions and readmissions for heart failure, and hospital deaths due to heart failure. The initiative included support for GPs and their practice teams to undertake audit of their current practice in managing heart failure, identifying patients with heart failure, an educational programme for patients with heart failure, and better access to diagnostic echocardiography. Prescribing of ACE inhibitors and loop diuretics increased by 18% and 27%, respectively, while prescribing of potassium-sparing diuretics decreased by 37% over a 2-year period. Readmission rates and deaths in hospital from heart failure decreased.

Managing patients with heart failure as a primary care team

The primary care team should develop a structured approach to managing patients with heart failure in their practice population (*see* Figure 5.1).

1 Identify and classify patients with heart failure.
   • Review those with a diagnosis of heart failure to check that the classification is correct.
   • Establish a heart failure disease register – preferably computerised with consistent use of Read coding (until Read coding is phased out and replaced by SNOMED).

2 Agree a protocol between general practice and the acute hospital with regard to the investigation and long-term management of patients with heart failure.
   • Develop this protocol for the district.
   • Establish a service which allows rapid access to echocardiography and/or cardiological opinion.
   • Encourage individual primary care teams to understand, own and adhere to the protocol.
3 Provide regular review and continuing care according to the practice protocol.
   • Give risk factor advice, particularly in relation to smoking cessation, physical activity, alcohol consumption and diet.
   • Advise on and treat raised blood pressure.
   • Immunise against influenza annually and immunise once against pneumococcus.
   • Control blood glucose and blood pressure levels in patients with diabetes.
   • Assess social needs and provision of long-term support.
   • Provide cardiac rehabilitation programmes.
   • Develop appropriate palliative care for end-stage heart failure.

Figure 5.1: Diagnostic algorithm for suspected heart failure in primary care (modified from North of England Evidence-Based Guideline Development Project[13,14]).

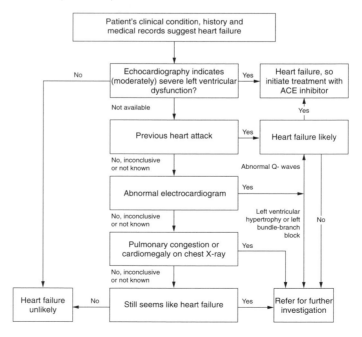

Reflection exercise

Exercise 9

Find out what the district-wide guidelines for heart failure are, if you do not know already.

Compare your practice protocol and any audit of your practice performance with the district guidelines or outcome data. Outcomes might include patients' quality of life, individual patients' functional capacity (e.g. the New York Heart Association functional capacity classification; *see* Box 5.1), prescribing data, adverse effects of treatment, mortality, hospital (re)admission rates, etc. How do you match up? Do you, your practice team or those advising you in your primary care organisation have any learning needs?

Now that you have completed this interactive reflection exercise, transfer the information to the relevant section about your learning needs in the empty template on pages 142–151 if you are working on your own personal development plan, or to the practice personal and professional development plan on pages 165–172 if you are working on a practice team learning plan. Don't forget to keep the evidence of your learning in your personal portfolio.

Further reading

Iqbal Z, Chambers R and Woodmansey P (2001) *Implementing the National Service Framework for Coronary Heart Disease for Primary Care*. Radcliffe Medical Press, Oxford.

This book provides comprehensive information about how to set up a heart failure register, create a practice protocol and familiarise oneself with the expectations of the National Service Framework for coronary heart disease for England with regard to heart failure.

References

1 Barton S (ed.) (2001) *Clinical Evidence. Issue 5.* BMJ Publishing Group, London.

2 Hobbs FDR (2000) Management of heart failure: evidence versus practice. Does current prescribing provide optimal treatment for heart failure? (Review article) *Br J Gen Pract.* **50**: 735–42.

3 Scottish Intercollegiate Guidelines Network (1999) *Diagnosis and Treatment of Heart Failure due to Left Ventricular Systolic Dysfunction.* SIGN Secretariat, Edinburgh.

4 Khunti K, Baker R and Grimshaw G (2000) Diagnosis of patients with chronic heart failure in primary care: usefulness of history, examination and investigations. *Br J Gen Pract.* **50**: 50–4.

5 Hopcroft K (2000) *The GP Guide to Secondary Care Investigations.* Radcliffe Medical Press, Oxford.

6 Collier J (ed.) (2000) Heart failure drugs: what's new? *Drug Ther Bull.* **38**: 25–7.

7 Hobbs FDR, Davis RC, McLeod S *et al.* (1998) Prevalence of heart failure in high-risk groups. *J Am Coll Cardiol.* **31 (Supplement 5)**: 85C (abstract).

8 The Heart Outcomes Prevention Evaluation (HOPE) Investigators (2000) Effects of an angiotensin-converting-enzyme inhibitor, ramipril, on cardiovascular events in high-risk patients. *NEJM.* **342**: 1445–53.

9 Evans D, Hood S and Taylor S (2000) Clinical effectiveness in the real world: lessons learned from a project to improve the management of patients with heart failure. *Clin Govern Bull.* **1**: 2–3.

10 Cleland JGF, McGowan J and Clark A (1999) The evidence for beta-blockers in heart failure equals or surpasses that for angiotensin-converting-enzyme inhibitors. *BMJ.* **318**: 824–5.

11 Clark A and Leland J (2000) Trials support use of beta-blockers in chronic heart failure. *Guidelines Pract.* **3**: 33–40.

12 Edinburgh Health Care Trust (1996) *Heart Manual.* Astley Ainslie Hospital, Edinburgh and Albert Gate Ltd, Grimsby.

13 Eccles M, Freemantle N, Mason JM and the North of England ACE-Inhibitor Guideline Development Group, North of England Evidence-Based Guideline Development Project (1998) Guideline for angiotensin-converting-enzyme inhibitors in primary care management of adults with symptomatic heart failure. *BMJ.* **316**: 1369–77.

14 Foord-Kelcey G (ed.) (2001) *Guidelines. Volume 13.* Medendium Group Publishing Ltd, Berkhamsted.

CHAPTER 6

Atrial fibrillation

What is atrial fibrillation?

This is a common heart rhythm disorder that occurs in about 2.5% of the general population of the UK and more frequently in older people. Nearly 10% of people aged 80–89 years have atrial fibrillation.[1-4]

In atrial fibrillation (AF), atrial activity is chaotic. The diagnosis is made from the ECG. AF may be paroxysmal or persistent, acute with spontaneous resolution or chronic.

Atrial fibrillation produces an inconsistent, irregular pulse. It may be symptomless, or may cause palpitations, breathlessness, ankle swelling and angina.

Atrial fibrillation is a very strong risk factor for stroke, as it predisposes to thromboembolism as a result of stasis and thrombus formation in the left atrium. Stroke is five to six times more common in people with AF than in patients of comparable age who are in sinus rhythm. About 15% of all patients who have experienced a stroke, and 2–8% of patients who have had a transient ischaemic attack, have atrial fibrillation. The stroke recurrence rate is 12% per year for a patient with atrial fibrillation.[3]

Acute atrial fibrillation may be self-limiting, and this is especially likely following acute myocardial infarction or after acute and excessive alcohol intake. Spontaneous cardioversion to a normal sinus rhythm occurs in nearly 50% of patients with paroxysmal or recent-onset atrial fibrillation.

Causes of atrial fibrillation

Cardiovascular causes

These include the following:

- valvular heart disease, such as mitral valve stenosis, regurgitation or valve prolapse (enquire about a history of rheumatic fever)
- hypertension
- ischaemic heart disease, including acute myocardial infarction
- cardiomyopathies
- congenital heart disease
- constrictive pericarditis
- post-cardiac surgery.

Other causes

These include the following:

- thyrotoxicosis
- acute illness, such as pneumonia
- pulmonary embolus
- excessive alcohol intake.

Investigations

ECG

P-waves are absent and there may be rapid irregular fibrillatory waves which vary in size, shape and timing, and widely spaced QRS complexes. The ECG may show that there has been a previous myocardial infarction or left ventricular hypertrophy secondary to hypertension.

A 24-hour ECG is needed if paroxysmal atrial fibrillation is suspected.

Chest X-ray

You will be looking for evidence of mitral stenosis, cardiomegaly and pulmonary oedema.

Blood tests

These will include the following:

- full blood count
- creatinine, urea and electrolytes
- thyroid function tests
- digoxin concentration if appropriate
- liver function tests if appropriate (e.g. if an alcohol binge is suspected as the cause of atrial fibrillation).

Echocardiography

An echocardiogram is used to determine whether there are any structural abnormalities in the heart which might be responsible for the atrial fibrillation, looking particularly at the left ventricular size and function, and left atrial size. It can detect atrial thrombus. The assessment by echocardiogram helps in the assessment of thrombo-embolic risk and the need for anticoagulation.

Treatment

Detection and treatment of the underlying cause is the first priority, so that hopefully sinus rhythm is restored spontaneously.

Controlling the heart rate[5,6]

Treatment should be instituted if the atrial fibrillation is impairing or threatening to impair cardiac function because the ventricular rate is so rapid. A ventricular rate above 90–100 beats per minute generally requires treatment.

- Digoxin can usually control the ventricular rate, although it may be ineffective during exercise. Overdose causes nausea and bradycardia (consult the *British National Formulary*[6] for more details). Impaired renal function and hypokalaemia can increase the serum digoxin concentration, so both should be monitored. Digoxin levels of 1.5–3.0 micrograms/L may indicate toxicity.

- Beta-blocker drugs such as atenolol and metoprolol are alternatives if the heart rate remains uncontrolled at rest or on exercise, despite digoxin.
- Rate-limiting calcium channel-blocking drugs, verapamil and diltiazem are other alternatives to digoxin.

Assessing the risk

The risk of stroke resulting from non-valvular atrial fibrillation is about 5% per year. Patients who are at highest risk of stroke include those aged over 75 years who have other risk factors, such as the following:

- diabetes
- hypertension
- past history of transient ischaemic attack or stroke
- valve disease
- heart failure
- thyroid disease.

Patients at moderate risk of stroke include those under 65 years of age with risk factors such as hypertension and diabetes. Also at moderate risk are individuals aged 65–75 years who do not have any high-risk factors.

People at low risk of stroke are those aged under 65 years with no history of embolism, hypertension, diabetes or other clinical risk factors.

Options for preventing thromboembolism[1–5,7]

Anticoagulation is more likely to be indicated in patients with valvular or myocardial disease, where the risk of stroke warrants it.

- High risk of stroke (12% annually): use warfarin (target international normalised ratio (INR) in the range 2.0–3.0).
- Moderate risk of stroke (8% annually): use aspirin or warfarin. Aspirin is recommended for high- or moderate-risk patients who decline warfarin or who are poor candidates for warfarin.
- Low risk of stroke (1% annually): use aspirin (75 mg once daily).

There have been five large randomised primary prevention trials which have demonstrated that anticoagulation with warfarin reduces the risk of stroke by 68%, compared with a 21% reduction in patients using aspirin. For those patients who have had a stroke, anticoagulation

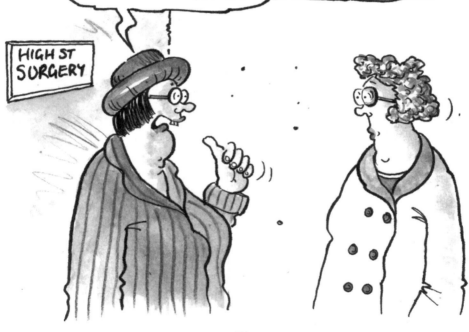

also reduces the risk of further strokes (i.e. as part of secondary prevention).[8]

The risk of intracranial haemorrhage increases with anticoagulation. Aim for an optimum INR for anticoagulation in non-valvular atrial fibrillation of between 2.0 and 3.0. This target should minimise the risk of intracranial haemorrhage whilst providing maximal thrombo-prophylaxis. In those over 75 years of age, a target INR of 1.6–2.5 is recommended as a better balance between risk and benefit.[8,9]

Box 6.1

The evidence for the trade-offs between benefits and harm asso-ciated with the use of anticoagulants and antiplatelet treatment in patients with atrial fibrillation continues to accumulate. Each person's treatment preferences should be considered too (*see* Box 6.2 below). Oral anticoagulation is currently widely used in preference to antiplatelet medication in patients with atrial fibrillation, to reduce the risk of cardiovascular mortality and morbidity. A systematic review of direct comparisons between long-term anticoagulation and antiplatelet treatment throws some doubt on current advice.[1] The study found no significant differ-ences between the two treatments in the prevention of fatal stroke and fatal or non-fatal cardiovascular events, but the findings were inconclusive. There was a difference of borderline significance for non-fatal stroke.[10] Larger research trials are needed to assess the long-term benefits and disadvantages of both approaches. Look out for future issues of *Clinical Evidence*[7] to keep you up to date as further research is published.

There is little evidence to support the use of dipyridamole, clopidogrel and ticlopidine as a substitute for warfarin in the prevention of stroke in patients with atrial fibrillation.

Contraindications to warfarin treatment include the following:

- an increased risk of bleeding from a coexisting medical condition (e.g. peptic ulcer)
- a tendency to falls
- interactions with other long-term drugs (consult the *British National Formulary*[6] for more information)
- likelihood of poor adherence to therapy.

The start of warfarin therapy should be delayed until at least 2 weeks after a cerebral embolic stroke has occurred.

> **Box 6.2** Patient preferences may not fit with the evidence[11]
>
> The use of anticoagulation for patients with atrial fibrillation is uncommon in the UK. Not only are many patients who are at high risk not prescribed warfarin, but as many as one-third of paients who are eligible for warfarin, according to established criteria, decline therapy after interviews in which the risks and consequences are explained.

Cardioversion

External electrocardioversion is given as a synchronised external direct current under general anaesthesia. Unless the atrial fibrillation has been present for less than 48 hours, the patient requires anticoagulation for at least 3 weeks before and at least 4 (some authorities recommend 26) weeks after the electrocardioversion. Amiodarone is sometimes given subsequently, to improve the likelihood of maintaining the sinus rhythm. The success rate varies for different centres, but is in the range 65–90%.

Pharmacological cardioversion is sometimes tried for atrial fibrillation of recent onset with intravenous or oral flecainide and propafenone for specific patients who have been anticoagulated as for electrical cardioversion. Because these drugs have potentially serious adverse effects, digoxin, beta-blocker and calcium-channel drugs (as described above) are usually preferred for long-term treatment.

Ablation therapy[12]

Ablation therapy is occasionally used for patients with atrial fibrillation who are very debilitated and in whom standard pharmacological therapy has failed or proved toxic. The treatment aims to destroy electrical conduction through the atrioventricular node. The patient is fitted with a permanent pacemaker and requires long-term anticoagulation.

We have only covered atrial fibrillation here as the most common type of cardiac arrhythmia, to demonstrate the extent of knowledge you might require in your everyday practice. You can use the same principles to learn more about best practice for other cardiac arrhythmias, such as atrial flutter, paroxysmal supraventricular tachycardia, ventricular tachycardia, etc.

Reflection exercises

Exercise 10

Review your practice protocol for atrial fibrillation (if you do not have a practice protocol, now is the time to write one) and what your practice team knows about diagnosis and management.

(i) Do you and your GP colleagues know and understand the stages in the protocol and criteria for treatment with thrombolytic and antiplatelet drugs?
    Discuss the protocol and implications for the practice over coffee.
(ii) Have you undertaken an audit of drug therapy – warfarin and digoxin – in the last 12 months?
    Why not do one now including all those who are regularly pre-scribed both drugs, and review whether patients taking these drugs should still be on treatment, or if other drugs may be interacting?

Exercise 11

How many people have you identified as having atrial fibrillation in your practice population?

How do the proportions compare with those described in this chapter? Do you need to redouble your efforts to identify individuals with atrial fibrillation from among your patients?

Now that you have completed these interactive reflection exer-cises, transfer the information to the relevant section about your learning needs in the empty template on pages 142–151 if you are working on your own personal development plan, or to the practice personal and professional development plan on pages 165–172 if you are working on a practice team learning plan. Don't forget to keep the evidence of your learning in your personal portfolio.

References

1 Lip GY and Lowe GD (1996) ABC of atrial fibrillation. *BMJ*. **312**: 45–9.
2 O'Kane P and Jackson G (2000) Atrial fibrillation: an update. *Update*. **17** February: 241–9.

3 Kamath S and Lip GY (2000) Managing cardiac arrhythmias. *Practitioner.* **244**: 568–73.

4 British Heart Foundation (2000) *Management of Atrial Fibrillation. Part 2.* Factfile 12/2000. British Heart Foundation, London.

5 Lancaster R and Carey P (2000) Atrial fibrillation. Top 100. *GP.* **21 July**: 42–3.

6 Mehta D (ed.) (2000) *British National Formulary.* British Medical Association and the Royal Pharmaceutical Society of Great Britain, London.

7 Barton S (ed.) (2001) *Clinical Evidence. Issue 5.* BMJ Publishing Group, London.

8 Hylek EM, Skates SJ, Sheehan MA *et al.* (1996) An analysis of the lowest effective intensity of prophylactic anticoagulation for patients with non-rheumatic atrial fibrillation. *NEJM.* **335**: 540–6.

9 Taylor FC, Cohen H and Ebrahim S (2001) Systematic review of long-term anticoagulation or antiplatelet treatment in patients with non-rheumatic atrial fibrillation. *BMJ.* **322**: 321–6.

10 Cobbe SM (1999) Atrial fibrillation in hospital and general practice: the Sir James McKenzie Centenary Consensus Conference. *Proc R Coll Physicians Edinburgh.* **29 (Supplement 6)**.

11 Howitt A and Armstrong D (1999) Implementing evidence-based medicine in general practice: audit and qualitative study of antithrombotic treatment for AF. *BMJ.* **318**: 1324–7.

12 British Heart Foundation (2001) *Ablation Therapy for Arrhythmias.* Factfile 1/2001. British Heart Foundation, London.

CHAPTER 7

Stroke

What is stroke?

A *stroke* is the sudden onset of clinical symptoms and signs of a focal, sometimes widespread, loss of cerebral function due to a vascular cause.

A *transient ischaemic attack* (TIA) is an acute loss of focal cerebral or monocular function with symptoms lasting for less than 24 hours.

Stroke is important because it is the third commonest cause of death in the developed world.[1] The annual incidence of stroke in developed countries is about two per 1000 members of the population, and the prevalence is about 5 per 1000 members of the population. The annual incidence of TIA is about 0.5 per 1000 members of the population.

Although a stroke can occur at any age, 50% of all strokes occur in people aged over 70 years. Most strokes[1] (about 80%) are due to the cutting off of the blood supply (ischaemic stroke). The artery becomes blocked by a thrombus that is either formed in that blood vessel or by an embolus that has broken off from a clot formed elsewhere. About 20% of strokes are caused by haemorrhage into or around the brain (subarachnoid haemorrhage).

About 10% of patients with an ischaemic stroke die within the first month and about 50% of the survivors will still have some disability after the first 6 months.[2] The disability will vary according to the part of the brain that has been affected.

The clinical picture

The commonest symptoms include the rapid onset of the following:

- numbness or weakness of the face, arm or leg, especially on one side
- confusion
- difficulty in speaking or understanding
- visual disturbance in one or both eyes

- difficulty in walking, loss of balance or co-ordination, or dizziness
- severe headache without a known cause.

Other less common symptoms include the following:

- a brief loss of consciousness, or a period of altered consciousness (confusion, coma, convulsions or 'passing out')
- the sudden onset within minutes or a few hours of nausea or vomiting, sometimes with a raised body temperature, but with a much more rapid onset than occurs with a viral infection.

Other symptoms and the signs present will vary according to the part of the brain that has been affected.

Right-hemisphere stroke

This often causes paralysis in the left side of the body (left hemiplegia). Spatial and perceptual problems lead to people misjudging distances (causing falls), and being unable to guide their hands accurately to tie their shoelaces, fasten buttons or pick objects up. They may place a book upside down to read it.

Alteration in judgement may be manifested in changes in behaviour. The patient may become more impulsive and be quite unaware of their disability. This can be dangerous if someone with a spatial or perceptual impairment tries to walk without help, or to drive a car.

The loss of visual field may cause the sufferer to ignore or forget objects or people on their left-hand side. This adds to the loss of short-term memory that often accompanies a stroke.

Left-hemisphere stroke

The loss of control over movement causes a right hemiplegia. As the left hemisphere controls speech and language, damage here can result in a variety of impairments, ranging from loss of the ability to find the right word for an object or person to a complete loss of speech (aphasia). The speech may become altered in content or type. Loss of understanding of words may frustrate any social interaction.

In contrast to right-hemisphere stroke sufferers, people with left-hemisphere strokes usually become slow and more cautious. They sometimes require constant reinforcement to complete any task, such as washing or eating. Loss of short-term memory, difficulty

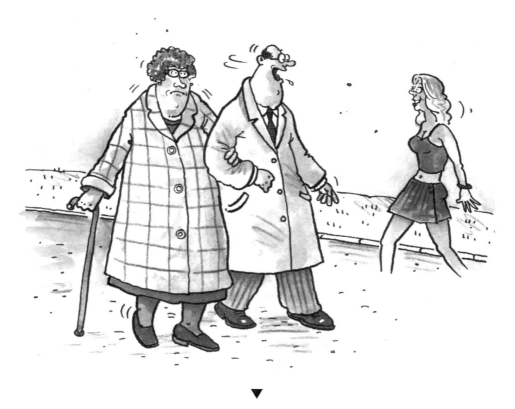

▼

'Loss of visual field may cause the sufferer to
ignore people on their left-hand side.'

in learning new information, and problems with conceptualisation and generalisation also occur.

Cerebellar stroke

Vascular events that affect the cerebellum cause abnormal reflexes in the head and trunk, with co-ordination and balance problems. Dizziness, nausea and vomiting can be distressing.

Brainstem strokes

This area of the brain controls the involuntary 'life-support' systems such as breathing, blood pressure and heart rate. A stroke in this part of the brain is often fatal. Eye movements, hearing, speech and swallowing are affected by injury to the brainstem. Hemiplegia or paraplegia may accompany these signs and symptoms, as the control from the hemispheres has to pass through the brainstem to other parts of the body.

Immediate assessment of the acute stroke

A full assessment of the patient requires both medical and multidisciplinary input (see Table 7.1).

Early referral to specialist support services and investigations improves the prognosis. Research shows that patients are more likely to be alive and living at home a year after the stroke if they are looked after by a specialised stroke team than if they are managed in general medical wards.[1]

Management by a specialised stroke team also reduces the length of time that is spent in hospital. The results of a systematic review of randomised controlled trials have been confirmed by observational studies in routine clinical settings.[1]

All stroke patients should be screened for swallowing difficulties by appropriately trained staff. This is usually done by observation of the patient being able to swallow plain water, recording the level of consciousness and noting whether any laryngeal abnormality is present. Immediate referral to a speech and language therapist for a more detailed assessment is necessary if there is any doubt about the ability to swallow normally. Inability to swallow carries a high risk of death.

Table 7.1 Initial assessment of acute stroke

Medical assessment	Nursing and PAM* assessment
Establishing from the history and examination that this is a vascular event	Assessment of the ability to swallow
Identifying the part of the brain that is affected	Establishing the extent and nature of functional impairment present
Determining whether the stroke is ischaemic or haemorrhagic	
Establishing the cause of the vascular event	
Determining whether other medical conditions coexist, and what effect they will have on the management	Determining what social problems the impairments will cause
Determining what facilities are needed to manage the patient effectively	

* Professions allied to medicine (e.g. physiotherapists, speech and language therapists, occupational therapists).

Investigations

Computerised tomography (CT)

CT brain scanning is useful for differentiating between haemorrhagic and ischaemic strokes if it is performed within 48 hours. Small bleeds can resolve rapidly and become impossible to differentiate from an infarct after a few days. CT scanning may also identify a non-stroke cause of the symptoms and signs (e.g. a brain tumour). An accurate diagnosis aids decision making about treatment and management.

Magnetic resonance imaging (MRI)

This investigation is more expensive and less readily available than CT scanning. In contrast to CT scanning, MRI is not so reliable for distinguishing between ischaemic and haemorrhagic causes in the first few days, but it can do so several weeks after the acute stroke. MRI is more reliable than CT scanning for identifying brainstem infarcts and bleeds into the posterior fossa.

Routine investigations

A full blood count, erythrocyte sedimentation rate, biochemical screen and lipid profile provide evidence of coexisting disease and a baseline for future management. A chest X-ray and electrocardiogram may reveal evidence of heart disease and an embolic source.

Other investigations

The clinical picture or the investigations may suggest other tests, such as the following:

- echocardiography – where heart disease is found or if there have been multiple episodes
- carotid Doppler ultrasound – after recovery from a stroke (or transient ischaemic attack) that was in the territory of the carotid artery and surgery is being considered
- other blood tests – especially in young patients, to determine whether there is an identifiable underlying increased risk of thrombosis (or of a bleeding disorder in a haemorrhagic stroke).

Immediate management of an acute stroke

Admission to hospital

Patients should normally be admitted to hospital, especially if any of the following are found:

- depressed level of consciousness
- fluctuating symptoms and signs
- difficulty in swallowing
- doubt about the diagnosis
- serious underlying disease
- suspicion of a haemorrhage, or if the patient is on anticoagulant treatment
- immobility, confusion, incontinence or adverse home circumstances.

If there is no agreed policy between primary and secondary care about referral or admission to hospital, you might consider how this could be set up. If the patient is not admitted to hospital, then urgent assessment is needed. In a few areas, trials have included a roving stroke care team that provides services at home, but urgent CT scanning (within 24 to 48 hours) still needs to be done. The Scottish Intercollegiate Guidelines Network (SIGN)[3] suggests that all patients who are looked after at home should be assessed at fast-track out-patient clinics as soon as possible after a minor stroke or transient ischaemic attack (TIA) has occurred. The risk of a further more serious stroke after a TIA is seven times higher than in the general population of the same age.

Drug therapy

Antiplatelet treatment with aspirin that is started within 48 hours of a stroke which has been confirmed to be ischaemic by CT scanning reduces the risk of death and dependence.[1] Some patients may benefit from thrombolytic therapy after an ischaemic stroke, but there is a risk of catastrophic intracerebral haemorrhage. It is not yet clear how to select which patients to treat.[1]

Other treatments, such as corticosteroids, nimodipine and other calcium antagonists, or haemodilution techniques, have not been shown to be helpful. Trials of other drugs are still under way.[1]

Do not reduce an elevated blood pressure in the acute phase of a stroke, as a number of trials have shown a poorer outcome when this was done.[1]

If a haemorrhagic stroke has been confirmed, correction of any coagulation defects is urgent, and, of course, patients should not be given aspirin.

Intracerebral haematomas may require surgical evacuation, especially if there is deterioration in the level of consciousness or there are signs of raised intracranial pressure. Patients with a cerebellar stroke may need urgent decompression of an acute hydrocephalus.

Complications following an acute stroke

Many of the deaths that occur in the first month after a stroke are due to immobility leading to conditions such as chest infections or pulmonary embolism.[4] Other complications can delay rehabilitation efforts (*see* Table 7.2).

Table 7.2 Frequency of complications after an acute stroke[5]

Complication	Frequency (%)
Falls	22
Pressure sores	18
Urinary tract infections	16
Chest infections	12
Depression	5
Confusion	5
Painful shoulder	4
Epileptic seizure	4
Deep venous thrombosis (DVT)	3
Pulmonary embolus	1

As mentioned above, chest infections are a common cause of death in the first few weeks after an acute stroke. Detection of swallowing problems and prevention of aspiration, as well as posture management and early mobilisation, are important preventive measures. Incontinence or incomplete bladder emptying are common after a stroke. Indwelling catheters make nursing and skin care easier but urinary tract infections are almost inevitable. Therefore other methods of dealing with incontinence should be explored.

Training everyone involved in patient handling may help to prevent shoulder pain. This includes the multidisciplinary team, the family and, where possible, the patient. Early mobilisation can also help in the prevention and treatment of shoulder pain, and in the prevention of a deep venous thrombosis (DVT), which will obviously be more likely to occur in immobile limbs. Good handling and frequent movement will also help to prevent pressure sores, soft tissue shortening and chest infections, as well as promoting recovery of motor control. Physiotherapy assessments help the planning of suitable interventions and the setting of realistic goals for recovery.

Depression is common in the first 3 months, occurring in about 25% of surviving patients,[6] and may adversely affect rehabilitation efforts.

Box 7.1

Mrs M attended her doctor several times with minor complaints, and seemed to be making much of them. When she was asked directly if anything else was worrying her, she told the doctor that her husband, who had been discharged from hospital six weeks earlier after a stroke, seemed to be doing less than he was when he had first come home, and kept shouting at her. Mr M agreed to talk to the community psychiatric nurse (CPN) after discussion with the physiotherapist whom he was still seeing. He had become clinically depressed after hearing that his daughter was moving house. As a retired builder, he had done much of the work on her previous house to get it just right for her. The CPN was able to help Mr M through his feelings of anger and despair that he would no longer be able to do the jobs around the house that he had taken such pride in before.

Patients with speech impairment have added psychosocial problems, and both patients and carers may become frustrated and angry. Speech and language therapists have an important role but, like other therapists, they are often in short supply.

Box 7.2

Mr W had always been the 'head of the household', and he and his wife had traditional, rigid roles before his stroke. His stroke had affected both his speech and his ability to calculate. After returning home, he became quite violent because he had to watch his wife learning how to pay the bills and he could not find the words to tell her what she should do. The speech and language therapist helped him by using intensive therapy and aids to communication, but Mr W remained very emotionally labile and impulsive. Fortunately for Mrs W, his lack of co-ordination meant that the missiles he directed at her rarely came anywhere near her, but the couple became increasingly socially isolated because of his behaviour.

Secondary prevention following an acute stroke

After an ischaemic stroke or TIA, aspirin should be continued. A low dose (75 mg daily) works just as well as higher doses while minimising side-effects. Aspirin can be given as a suppository if the patient has swallowing problems. Other antiplatelet drugs have not been shown to be any more effective than aspirin, but dipyridamole has a similar effect to aspirin, and may have an additive effect in combination.[3]

Anticoagulation therapy in patients with atrial fibrillation may be indicated, but a recent systematic review[7] casts doubt on the relative merits of anticoagulant and antiplatelet long-term therapies.

There is little clear evidence for the effectiveness of risk reduction advice,[1] but it seems sensible to stop smoking, and to control diabetes, hypertension and hyperlipidaemia.

Box 7.3

A general practice asked for help from a voluntary organisation that had a minibus adapted for wheelchairs with a rear-entry rise-and-fall step. Several patients with walking difficulties were transported to the 'stop smoking' group run by the practice nurse, who was also able to arrange for these patients to have other health screening while they were at the health centre premises.

Rehabilitation following an acute stroke

As with all chronic illnesses, a well-maintained stroke register will enable the practice team to offer effective follow-up care and regularly review all those identified on the disease register.

Rehabilitation should be started as soon as the patient's condition allows.[8] A multidisciplinary team that is interested in stroke helps to maximise recovery of function. Good team networking and management involves the following:[8]

- an identified member of the team to act as a key worker with the patient and carer
- full discussion with the patient and carer about the stroke, its management and expectations with regard to the outcome
- good documentation, so that consistent information and management are provided by all of the team members
- information given to patients and carers both verbally and in writing
- rehabilitation aims discussed and agreed by all members of the team, including the patient and carer
- continued assessment that takes note of the patient's changing needs, as reductions in impairment can be achieved even a year after the stroke.

The Scottish Intercollegiate Guidelines Network (SIGN) guidelines[8] emphasise the need for education and training for the whole multidisciplinary team, including nurses, physiotherapists, occupational therapists, speech and language therapists, and a doctor with a special interest in stroke. Other professionals may be needed, such as a psychologist or dietitian. Voluntary societies can give patients and carers much-needed support and help (*see* list of useful addresses at the end of this chapter).

Discharge from hospital should be well planned. An assessment in the patient's own home by an occupational therapist who rates the ability of the patient to manage tasks at home can be very helpful.[8] Collaboration between a hospital-based stroke care team and the primary care health and social services teams that will take over the patient's management seems an obvious – but often neglected – step before discharge home.

It is common sense that patients should not be discharged home before the services that they need are in place, and if this is happening then it indicates an urgent need to review local policies.

Box 7.4

One Saturday morning, the doctor was enraged to find that one of his patients had been discharged from hospital on a Friday afternoon to an empty house devoid of food. On investigation, it appeared that a changeover of hospital staff had resulted in a lack of communication about the arrangements, and the patient had been discharged on the Friday instead of the following Monday. It had not been appreciated that the patient was unaware of his limitations, and that he had assumed that he would be able to walk to the local shops as he had done before admission.

Many of the rehabilitation efforts, such as speech and language therapy and physiotherapy, which were started in hospital will need to be continued once the patient has gone home. It is very important that the key member of the multidisciplinary team co-ordinates the activities of all of these efforts, and a formal plan may be the best way to achieve the most effective care without duplication of effort.[8] A patient-held record may be one way to ensure that everyone has the necessary information, but constant reinforcement is necessary to ensure that the relevant staff always complete it. Often the patient or principal carer is the best person to remind the team members to record what they have done and what is planned, as well as their contact arrangements.

Help with daily living

Regaining some measure of independence is an important factor in recovery. Nurses, occupational therapists and other team members can give advice on adaptive devices that make completing everyday tasks easier. Grab bars in the bathroom or toilet, a raised toilet seat, bath or shower seats, and an electric toothbrush and shaver all help with independent care. Even quite simple advice can make a difference.

Box 7.5

Although Mr S could now have a shower, he was reluctant to do this on his own. His key nurse discovered that he could not dry himself well enough with his small towels, and that he found the large bath sheets too heavy to manage. His son bought him some long light roller towels that he found much easier to manage, and he was pleased that he was now able to have a shower when he wanted, not only when the nursing assistant could help him with one.

Kitchen modifications and aids help with meal preparation and eating. Structural alterations to the home may need to be made. Widening doorways to accommodate walking with a frame, or fitting a stair rail on both sides so that the good hand can be used, can make an enormous difference to mobility.

Box 7.6

When Mrs K returned home after her stroke, she and her daughter worked through her wardrobe, adapting those clothes that Mrs K could manage on her own, and discarding those that she could not. All the 'over-the-head' garments and those fastening at the back were set aside for the charity shop, and Velcro replaced the zips and buttons on the clothes that were retained. Some smart stretchy 'leisure suits' with easy large armholes completed the new image of this fiercely independent and fashion-conscious woman.

Simple common sense alterations to the way in which things are done can help patients with memory loss. A large calendar showing the date and day (changed daily by the carers!), boards on which to write reminders or pin notes, and keeping frequently used items in the same cupboard or drawer which is labelled with a list of the contents can all help.

Driving

After a stroke or TIA, patients should not drive for at least a month, or until clinical recovery is satisfactory. The Driver and Vehicle Licensing Agency should be notified.

Patients may be unaware of their disability, especially if they have had a right-hemisphere stroke, and can often cause their relatives considerable distress by insisting that they can drive safely.

Ethical issues

The healthcare team may be faced with ethical dilemmas about the treatment of severely impaired stroke sufferers. There may be issues concerning feeding, adequate hydration, artificial ventilation or treatment of infections. Consensus decisions should only be taken after full and informed discussion by the healthcare team and relatives. The decisions need to be clearly communicated to everyone involved in the care of the patient. Emotional support for both staff and relatives should be available when distressing decisions have to be made.

Useful addresses and websites

National Electronic Library for Stroke

This virtual branch library will contain information for the following:

- people who want to reduce their risk of stroke
- people who have had a stroke, and their carers
- primary care professionals
- specialists in stroke care
- public health professionals and managers.

Website: www.nlm.nih.gov/medlineplus/stroke.html

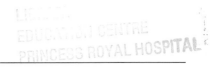

This site will be under construction until 2001. It will contain:

- stroke guidelines
- a patients' version linked to NHS Direct On-line
- links to SIGN, Stroke Cochrane, the British Association of Stroke Physicians, controlled trials register and patients' organisations.

Stroke

A list of local helplines for the Stroke Association, as well as leaflets and information, is available.

The Stroke Association, Stroke House, Whitecross Street, London EC1Y 8JJ. Tel: 020 7566 0300.

Website: www.stroke.org.uk

Different Strokes Charity for young stroke survivors

Contact: Donal O'Kelly, Different Strokes, Sir Walter Scott House, 2 Broadway Market, London E8 4QJ.

Email: different@strokes.demon.co.uk

Acute Stroke Toolbox

Although based in the USA, this contains much useful information for patients, carers and team members.

Website: www.stroke-site.org

Reflection exercises

Exercise 12

Do you know the mortality and morbidity rates for stroke in your district?

Have you any idea how those rates compare with national statistics? Do you know how well patients from different socio-economic groups fare? If you do, note down the local rates in your personal or practice learning plan to justify why you are focusing on learning more about stroke. If you do not know these statistics, then find out more from your local public health department.

Exercise 13

Review the patient literature you have on diet, smoking, body mass index and weight loss, alcohol consumption and physical activity.

How does the literature compare with the up-to-date recommendations given in this chapter? Ask patients who are at risk of heart disease or stroke, of different ages and backgrounds, to look at your patient literature and tell you whether it is appropriate – easy to read and relevant to them. Update your patient educational literature accordingly. Find out which self-help groups might supply more appropriate literature, or download material from suitable websites and photocopy it.

Now that you have completed these interactive reflection exercises, transfer the information to the relevant section about your learning needs in the empty template on pages 142–151 if you are working on your own personal development plan, or to the practice personal and professional development plan on pages 165–172 if you are working on a practice team learning plan. Don't forget to keep the evidence of your learning in your personal portfolio.

References

1 Barton S (ed.) (2001) *Clinical Evidence. Issue 5.* BMJ Publishing Group, London.

2 Bamford J, Sandercock P, Dennis M *et al.* (1990) A prospective study of acute cerebrovascular disease in the community: the Oxfordshire Community Stroke Project 1981–86. *J Neurol Neurosurg Psychiatry.* **53**: 16–22.

3 Scottish Intercollegiate Guidelines Network (1997) *Management of Patients with Stroke. Part 1.* SIGN Guideline No. 13. Scottish Intercollegiate Guidelines Network, Edinburgh.

4 Bamford J, Sandercock P, Dennis M *et al.* (1990) The frequency, causes and timings of death in the first 30 days of a first stroke: the Oxfordshire Community Stroke Project 1981–86. *J Neurol Neurosurg Psychiatry.* **53**: 824–9.

5 Davenport RJ, Dennis MS, Wellwood I *et al.* (1996) Complications after acute stroke. *Stroke.* **27**: 415–20.

6 Astrom M, Adolfsoson R and Asplund K (1993) Major depression in stroke patients. *Stroke.* **24**: 976–82.

7 Taylor FC, Cohen H and Ebrahim S (2001) Systematic review of long-term anticoagulation or antiplatelet treatment in patients with non-rheumatic atrial fibrillation. *BMJ.* **322**: 321–6.

8 Scottish Intercollegiate Guidelines Network (1998) *Management of Patients With Stroke. Part 4.* SIGN Guideline No. 24. Scottish Intercollegiate Guidelines Network, Edinburgh.

CHAPTER 8

Prevention of cardiovascular disease

Preventing cardiovascular disease is a major priority for those working in primary care. It is worth investing a huge effort because so much cardiovascular morbidity and mortality is preventable.

Primary prevention

Primary prevention is the long-term management of people at increased risk but with no evidence of cardiovascular disease. This includes the many adults who are at increased risk and have atheroma but no symptoms or obvious signs of vascular disease.[1]

Primary prevention of cardiovascular disease can be instituted as a population approach, or targeted at individuals in high-risk groups. The population approach is a long-term strategy which incorporates work on the wider economic and social determinants of ill health. Policies for reducing smoking, promoting healthy eating and physical activity and reducing obesity are targeted at the whole population by the NHS, local authorities, the education sector, etc. Reducing the whole population's risk levels by just a small amount can actually have more effect on overall morbidity and mortality than targeted approaches for high-risk individuals.

Secondary prevention

Secondary prevention is the long-term management of patients with existing vascular disease, and it aims to slow the progression of their vascular disease. Target groups are those people who already have heart disease, such as angina or myocardial infarction, or who have undergone revascularisation by angioplasty or coronary artery bypass grafting (CABG). Patients with cardiovascular disease such as transient ischaemic attacks (TIAs), stroke and peripheral vascular disease are also included.[1]

The aims of secondary prevention in modifying risk factors are long term, and the associated lifestyle changes are difficult to achieve and sustain.

Prioritising prevention

Primary care should focus on those who are at greatest risk of CHD and stroke. The top priority is secondary prevention for patients with established coronary heart disease or other major atherosclerotic disease. When secondary prevention has been instituted for all suitable patients, the next priority is primary prevention for those at risk. These individuals should be managed with a staged approach starting with those who have an absolute coronary heart disease risk of at least 30% over 10 years – that is, there is at least a 3 in 10 chance that they will have a major coronary event in the ensuing 10 years. When this group is receiving primary prevention, move to target those with an absolute risk of at least 15% of a major coronary event over 10 years as described in Box 8.2.[2]

It is well accepted that a reduction in hypertension leads to a reduced likelihood of stroke. Stroke is unusual in an individual without at least one risk factor for vascular disease.

The calculation of risk is based on age, gender, smoking status, presence or absence of diabetes, systolic blood pressure and the ratio of total cholesterol to HDL cholesterol.

Treating high-risk individuals

In people with a risk as low as 6%, interventions with drugs can reduce the risk of coronary heart disease events and deaths from all causes. Currently, if all individuals with this level of risk were identified and offered interventions, the enormous drain on the resources of the NHS could not be justified.[3]

> **Box 8.1**
>
> Using the higher priority of at least a 30% 10-year risk threshold for a practice of 10 000 patients, 293 individuals of all ages would require secondary prevention, and 56 individuals aged 35–69 years would be eligible for primary prevention.

The Joint British Recommendations on prevention of coronary heart disease in general practice recommend this staged approach (see Box 8.2).

> **Box 8.2** Summary of the Joint British Recommendations on the prevention of coronary heart disease (CHD) in general practice[2,4]
>
> *First priority: patients with established coronary heart disease or other atherosclerotic disease (i.e. secondary prevention)*
>
> - Relevant lifestyle changes: stopping smoking, increasing exercise, eating healthier food.
> - Blood pressure controlled (to levels below 140/85 mmHg).
> - In diabetes: optimal control of blood glucose, and blood pressure reduced to 140/80 mmHg or below; reduce total cholesterol concentration to less than 5.0 mmol/L and LDL cholesterol to less than 3.0 mmol/L.
> - Cardioprotective drug treatment for selected patients: aspirin, ACE inhibitors, beta-blockers, statins.
>
> *Second priority: patients without known coronary heart disease or other atherosclerotic disease (i.e. primary prevention)*
>
> There are three groups to be identified and managed in a staged approach – the group with the highest risk first. All groups should be given relevant lifestyle advice as described above.
>
> *1 Absolute CHD risk of at least 30% or more over 10 years*
> - Blood pressure controlled to levels to 140/85 mmHg or below.
> - Reduce total cholesterol concentration to less than 5.0 mmol/L and LDL cholesterol to less than 3.0 mmol/L.
> - In diabetes: optimal control of blood glucose, and blood pressure reduced to 140/80 mmHg or below.
> - Aspirin therapy if the patient is aged over 50 years and hypertensive, male, or both.

> 2 *Absolute CHD risk of at least 15% or more over 10 years*
> - Target progressively more patients and intervene as described above.
>
> 3 *Absolute CHD risk of less than 15% over 10 years*
> - Drug treatment is not required unless there is severe hypertension (over 160/100 mmHg), associated target organ damage or familial hyperlipidaemia.

The main risk factors for coronary heart disease

Fixed factors

These include the following:

- increasing age
- male gender
- family history (i.e. coronary heart disease before the age of 55 years in men and before the age of 65 years in women)
- other vascular diseases (e.g. stroke).

Modifiable/lifestyle factors

These include the following:

- smoking
- diet high in saturated fats
- diet low in fruit and vegetables
- excessive alcohol consumption
- physical inactivity.

Physiological/biological factors

These include the following:

- raised levels of total cholesterol and low-density lipoprotein
- sustained hypertension
- low levels of high-density lipoprotein
- high levels of plasma triglycerides
- diabetes

- obesity
- thrombogenic factors.

Box 8.3 Better health the more low-risk factors you have in your lifestyle[5]

'The big question, though, is whether combining all the different aspects of healthy living makes a substantial difference to health outcomes. If (you) were to give up smoking, start drinking (within recommended limits of alcohol), lose weight, eat properly and take some exercise, would it make any difference?'

The answer from one study of 122 000 female nurses aged 30 to 55 years was that a low-risk-factor lifestyle reduces the likelihood of a heart attack or stroke by about 80% over a period of 14 years or so.

Tools to assist measurement of risk

There is a range of charts and tables based on the Framingham data, as well as numerous types of software which calculate risk in the clinical setting.[6] Risk charts include the following:

- The Sheffield Table
- New Zealand Guidelines
- The Joint British Chart.

Problems with risk predictors include the following:

- risk predictions can be flawed when some of the variables are at their extremes
- family history is not included in the calculations, and therefore a positive family history may increase the risk above that indicated
- the charts underestimate the risks for individuals with familial hypercholesterolaemia
- the charts underestimate the risk for British Asians and those on low incomes.

Age

Elderly people have the same risk factors for coronary heart disease as the general population, although the association between risk factors and CHD may be less strong. As CHD is much more common in the elderly, they are as likely to benefit from preventive measures as younger people, if not more so.

Controlling hypertension is probably the most important modifiable risk factor for CHD in elderly people.

Gender

Very few trials have examined the risk factor status, intervention and outcomes in women. Many of the risk assessment tools extrapolate the results from trials including extrapolation of data from men to women. Although the overall treatment rates have improved in both men and women with CHD, women are still not prescribed drugs as often as men.[7]

Important gender differences and similarities include the following:

- higher rates of obesity and diabetes and higher total cholesterol levels in women aged over 55 years
- more frequent hypertension in women aged over 65 years than in men of similar age
- the onset of CHD in women lags behind that in men by about 10 years
- women under 65 years of age have one-third of the CHD mortality rate for men of a similar age
- women more commonly present with angina and men more commonly present with myocardial infarction
- women are as likely as men to reinfarct after a myocardial infarction; some studies have suggested that there is a poorer prognosis for women post-myocardial infarction.
- women are at least as likely to benefit from lipid-lowering drug therapy as men.

Minority ethnic groups

People from South Asia living in the UK have a much greater (about 50% higher) risk of developing coronary heart disease than white people living in the UK, while individuals of African-Caribbean descent living in the UK have a much lower risk (up to 50% less), but their risk of hypertension is higher.

In a recent survey in England, Pakistani and Bangladeshi men were found to have rates of cardiovascular disease about 60–70% higher than those for men of the same age and sex in the general population,[8] and the comparative rates for Pakistani and Bangladeshi women were almost as high.

Diabetes

Diabetes increases the risk of developing heart disease by up to fivefold, and heart disease is one of the most important causes of death among people with diabetes. Those with diabetes are also more likely to suffer from hypertension, hyperlipidaemia, heart failure and cardiogenic shock.[9,10]

Good control of blood sugar levels (e.g. keeping HbA_{1c} levels below 7.0%) will reduce the microvascular complications of diabetes. Modification of risk factors, particularly smoking, hyperlipidaemia and high blood pressure (e.g. ideally to 140/80 mmHg or less) is critical.[11]

There is a high absolute risk of cardiovascular disease in patients with diabetes, so there is a greater benefit from lipid-lowering therapy in people with diabetes compared with individuals without diabetes for a given cholesterol/HDL ratio.[12] There is some evidence to suggest that the available risk assessment methods may underestimate CHD risk in patients with type 1 diabetes. It seems as if the HDL in type 1 diabetes does not confer the same degree of protection against CHD as it does in people without diabetes. Therefore lipid-lowering therapy should be considered at a lower risk threshold in patients with diabetes.

Familial hypercholesterolaemia

Familial hypercholesterolaemia is an autosomal-dominant condition that affects about 1 in 500 of the UK population. Single-gene disorders such as familial hypercholesterolaemia may cause coronary heart disease at a young age. Genetic testing is complicated by ethical problems with regard to the commercial interest of insurance companies in predicting risk and weighting insurance premiums accordingly. Research into the genetic basis of coronary heart disease may lead to gene therapy.

Patients with this condition need to be treated aggressively with dietary advice and lipid-lowering therapy. Referral to a specialist clinic is recommended.

Targeting lifestyle to prevent cardiovascular disease

Figure 8.1 represents the cycle through which an individual must progress before they make changes to the lifestyle factors that you are targeting as a health professional. You will need to refine your approach depending on whether the person has no plans to change, is still contemplating whether to make the change, or is preparing to change (e.g. to give up smoking). They may need help in maintaining the change to prevent a relapse occurring subsequently.

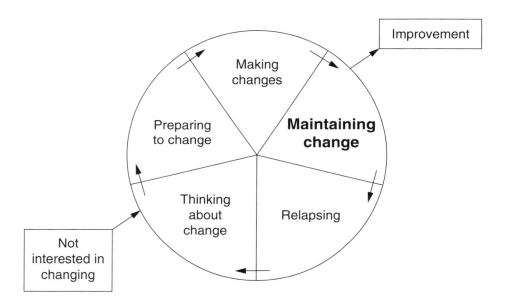

Figure 8.1: The process of change.

Cholesterol lowering by diet[1,6,9,13,14]

Blood lipids can be divided into different components, namely low-density-lipoprotein (LDL) cholesterol, high-density-lipoprotein (HDL) cholesterol and triglycerides. Low levels of HDL and high levels of LDL are associated with an increased risk of CHD. The ratio of total LDL cholesterol to HDL cholesterol is often used to assess the risk of CHD. In countries where the average cholesterol levels of the population are low, CHD rates tend to be low as well. The link between cholesterol level and future risk of CHD is continuous (i.e. there is no threshold above which CHD risks begin to increase). Thus lower levels of cholesterol are associated with a lower risk of CHD.

People who have recently had a myocardial infarction are more likely to be motivated to follow strict diets. However, research has not found any significant change in the overall coronary heart disease mortality following dietary interventions alone in high-risk patients. One explanation for this might be that dietary interventions often substitute total fat or carbohydrate, which reduces the levels of HDL cholesterol as well as LDL cholesterol. If the LDL/HDL ratio is unaffected, the magnitude of the coronary heart disease risk also remains unaffected. Therefore it is important to lower CHD risk rather than focusing exclusively on reduction of the cholesterol level.

Increased intake of oily fish and a trial of a Mediterranean diet have both been shown to reduce CHD mortality after a heart attack without affecting the cholesterol levels. The use of these interventions in the general population or in those at lower risk of CHD has not been tested.

Box 8.4 Fish on Fridays

As part of the Physicians' Health Study, male US physicians aged 40 to 84 years completed a questionnaire on the types of fish they ate and how often. They were followed up for 13 years. Eating fish at least once a week reduced the risk of sudden cardiac death by 52% (but with wide 95% confidence limits of 4–76%).[15] There was no effect on myocardial infarction or other cardiovascular disease endpoints. The authors concluded that eating fish improved a person's likelihood of surviving a heart attack. It did not matter what type of fish was eaten, and eating it more than once a week conferred no extra benefit. They postulated that the effect might be due to an anti-arrhythmic action of fish fatty acids.

Studies of cholesterol-lowering interventions mediated by a population approach have shown only small changes in cholesterol levels, with the overall reduction being around 1–5%. Although such a reduction is almost insignificant for an individual patient, it equates to a theoretical reduction in coronary heart disease mortality of up to 10% at a population level. In the UK this would represent the avoidance of 6000 deaths per year in people aged under 75 years.

Research has shown that garlic, oats and soya have a cholesterol-lowering effect. However, many of these research trials were small and

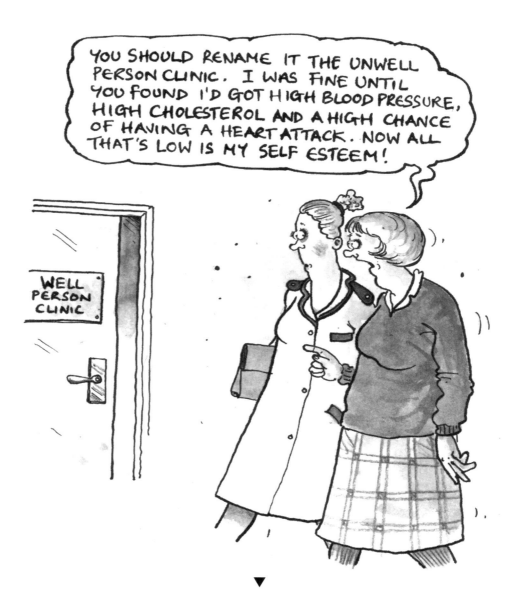

of relatively short duration, and therefore the results obtained are difficult to interpret.

Increased consumption of fruit and vegetables may also be protective against CHD. Foods (e.g. margarines) that are enriched with stanol esters or plant sterols also reduce cholesterol concentrations in those consuming an average cholesterol diet, but are not as effective in those on a low-fat diet.

Overweight and obesity

Being overweight is associated with raised blood pressure, raised blood cholesterol levels, low levels of physical activity, and glucose intolerance/non-insulin-dependent diabetes.

About 45% of men and 34% of women in the UK are overweight (body mass index (BMI) 25–30), and an additional 16% of men and 18% of women are obese (BMI >30). Around 15% of boys and girls are overweight, while an additional 1.5% are obese.[9,16]

No trials have been undertaken to assess the effect of weight reduction in secondary prevention, and therefore it is not known whether obesity is an independent risk factor. However, weight reduction should become part of secondary prevention management plans because of the adverse effect of obesity on other risk factors, the aim being to achieve body mass indices of less than 25 if possible.

Reductions in dietary salt content lead to reduced hypertension and thus reduced CHD risk.

Alcohol[16]

In the UK, 28% of men and 13% of women consume more alcohol than is recommended (a maximum of 14 units per week for women and 21 units for men), and 42% of young men and 27% of young women (aged 16–24 years) are estimated to drink more alcohol than the recommended limits. The proportion of women who drink more than the recommended amount is three times as high in professional groups as in unskilled groups in the general population.

Light to moderate drinkers have a lower CHD mortality than heavy drinkers. The British Heart Foundation recommends that alcohol in moderation may be beneficial for patients with established heart disease. However, a higher alcohol intake by the population in general has enormous adverse social and health consequences.

Box 8.5 Summary of advice on healthy living for individuals[5]

1 Eat whole-grain foods (bread, rice or pasta) four times a week.
2 Do not smoke, and give up if you do. Nicotine replacement (patches, gum or inhalers) may help some people to give up smoking altogether. There are no completely safe levels of smoking, but smoking less reduces the risk of cancer, heart or respiratory disease. Cut down to less than 5 cigarettes a day, and go for long periods in the day without smoking.
3 Eat at least 5 portions of vegetables and fruit a day, especially tomatoes (including ketchup), red grapes, and salad all year.
4 You could use Benecol instead of butter or margarine. It does reduce cholesterol levels, and reducing cholesterol will reduce the risk of heart attack and stroke even in those whose cholesterol level is not particularly high.
5 Reduce visible fat on meat and in gravy, and pare down the quantity of butter or margarine that you use, as an alternative to substituting with Benecol, etc.
6 Drink alcohol regularly within the recommended limits. The type of alcohol probably does not matter too much, but the equivalent of a couple of glasses of wine a day or a couple of beers is a good thing.
7 Eating fish once a week will not prevent you from having a heart attack, but it will reduce the likelihood of your dying from it by 50%.
8 Take a multivitamin tablet containing at least 200 micrograms of folate every day. This can substantially reduce the likelihood of heart disease in some individuals.
9 Walking a mile a day or taking reasonable exercise three times a week (enough to make you sweat or glow) will substantially reduce the risk of heart disease.
10 Your body mass index should be below 25. If you are overweight, lose the excess weight.

Physical activity

Two out of three men (64%) and three out of four women (76%) lead sedentary lives. Only 31% of men and 20% of women are active enough to gain some protection against coronary heart disease.

Physical activity is strongly associated with a lower risk of coronary heart disease. The largest reductions in risk are in individuals who were previously sedentary or moderately active, compared with modest risk reductions in those who were already vigorously active. Brisk walking or heavy gardening are particularly effective, especially if sustained for long periods.

Cardiac exercise rehabilitation following myocardial infarction has been shown to reduce all causes of mortality by 24%. All patients with heart disease who have no contraindications to exercise should take regular aerobic exercise at least three times a week for 20–30 minutes.[1]

Smoking[17–22]

Smoking is the single largest cause of preventable illness and premature death in the UK. An estimated 13 million adults in the UK are smokers. Smoking rates have fallen steadily for the last two decades, except for the last two to three years, when rates have fluctuated. About 28% of men and 26% of women are currently smokers.

Smoking is more common in lower socio-economic groups. Around 15% of men with professional jobs are smokers, compared with 45% of men in unskilled jobs. Smoking is more common in North-West England and in Scotland (31% and 30% of adults, respectively), compared with 24% of men who live in South-West England who are smokers.

Box 8.6 Smoking kills

Smoking kills around six times more people in the UK than road and other accidents, murders and manslaughter, suicide, poisoning, overdose and HIV added together.

Brief advice given by GPs for an average period of three minutes may only lead to 2–3% of smokers stopping smoking, but if this was replicated in the whole population, the 2–3% of people quitting smoking would translate into thousands of ex-smokers and enormous health benefits.

Intermediate-level smoking cessation services are 'smoking cessation support services based around general practice, and can involve either one-to-one or group support led by a member of the primary care team (e.g. a health visitor).' This service can be shared between practices.[23]

Specialist smoking cessation clinics take referrals of smokers who require more intensive or specialist help.[23] Specialist smoking cessation services:

- offer group support, but also provide support on an individual basis if necessary
- are manned by practitioners trained in smoking cessation techniques
- offer nicotine replacement therapy free to those exempt from pre-scription charges
- provide a variety of self-help materials.

Group programmes seem to be more effective than self-help pro-grammes. However, there is little evidence that group therapy is more effective than individual counselling of a similar intensity. The overall quit rate, including the background placebo quit rate in smokers' clinics, is estimated to be around 10%. A combination of pharmacotherapy and motivational support has the best success rate.

Table 8.1 An estimate of the relative effectiveness of various smoking interventions in the 'real world' rather than with highly motivated volunteers and staff [24]

Intervention	Percentage still abstinent after 12 months
Will-power alone	3%
Self-help materials (e.g. audiotapes, videos, booklets)	4%
Pharmacotherapy bought from a pharmacy	6%
Smokers' clinic but no pharmacotherapy	10%
Smokers' clinic plus pharmacotherapy	20%

Summary of effectiveness of interventions to help people stop smoking[25]

- Advice from doctors, structured interventions from nurses, and individual and group counselling are effective.
- Generic self-help materials are no better than brief advice, but are more effective than doing nothing. Personalised materials are more effective than standard materials.
- All forms of nicotine replacement are effective.
- Bupropion and nortriptyline have been shown to increase quit rates in a small number of trials.
- The usefulness of clonidine is limited by its side-effects.
- Anxiolytics and lobeline are ineffective.
- The effectiveness of aversion therapy, necamylamine, acupuncture, hypnotherapy and exercise is uncertain.

Nicotine replacement therapy (NRT) weans the addicted smoker off nicotine by a controlled reduction in intake and a subsequent reduction in withdrawal symptoms. NRT is available in the following forms:

- chewing gum
- transdermal patches
- nasal spray
- inhalers
- tablets.

All of the commercially available forms of NRT appear to be effective and increase quit rates by one and a half times to twofold.

Bupropion seems to be more effective than nicotine replacement therapy in smoking cessation. Box 8.7 lists the indications for its use. The evidence shows that:

> 'Oral bupropion is a non-nicotine preparation recently marketed as an aid to help stop smoking. It is available on the NHS as a prescription-only medicine. When used in a specialist setting and in conjunction with regular counselling, bupropion is at least twice as effective as placebo in helping patients to stop smoking. However, it is not clear what contribution the specialist setting makes to this outcome. Preliminary results suggest that bupropion is possibly more effective than a nicotine skin patch . . . but there are no published data on how bupropion compares with other forms of NRT.'[26]

Insomnia and dry mouth are common. Bupropion is contraindicated in patients who suffer from epilepsy, as it can cause seizures.

Box 8.7 Bupropion: indications for use

Bupropion is indicated for smokers if they:

- are motivated to quit
- have nicotine dependence
- have access to motivational support.

Indications of nicotine dependency include:

- smoking within 20 minutes of waking
- smoking regularly throughout the day
- smoking more than 15 cigarettes a day
- withdrawal symptoms on attempts to quit smoking.

The safety and efficacy of bupropion have not been evaluated for people under the age of 18 years.

Figure 8.2: Smoking cessation – protocol for intervention by GP or community nurse (modified from Fowler, 2000[27]).

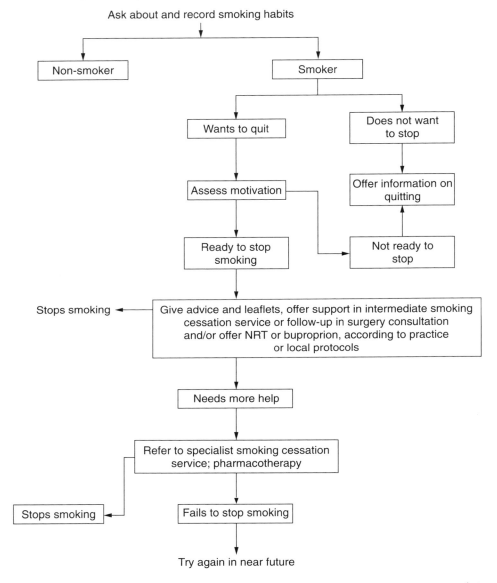

Establish smoking cessation services in your practice as suggested in Figure 8.2. Studies indicate that patients with coronary heart disease will reduce their risk of further fatal and non-fatal events by up to 50% over 2 years by giving up smoking. Those who continue to smoke are at up to three times higher risk of death compared with those who have stopped.

Smoking also reduces the prevalence of angina following a heart attack. Patients with angina who continue to smoke double their risk of subsequent cardiac events.

Pharmacological interventions to prevent cardiovascular disease

Antiplatelet therapy[1,28]

Antiplatelet therapy, when used for secondary prevention of myocardial infarction, regardless of age, gender, or the presence or absence of diabetes or hypertension, reduces the risk of:

- vascular death by one-sixth
- non-fatal myocardial infarction by one-third
- non-fatal stroke by one-third.

Aspirin is associated with an overall reduction in myocardial infarction, stroke or vascular death of 25%. Different aspirin dose regimens have similar benefits. Low-dosage aspirin (75 mg per day) reduces cardio-vascular risk in well-controlled hypertensive patients who have cardio-vascular complications or high-risk factors.

Beta-blocker drugs

Beta-blocker treatment reduces total mortality, sudden death and reinfarction rates following myocardial infarction. The beneficial effects last as long as the treatment continues. The benefits of long-term beta-blockade result in a 20% reduction in risk of death, a 25% reduction in risk of reinfarction and a 30% reduction in risk of sudden death (*see* Chapter 4 for further details).

Lipid-lowering drugs[1,6,9,29,30]

There have been two randomised controlled primary prevention trials involving pravastatin and lovastatin. Both of these trials showed significant reductions in cardiac event rates of around one-third. There have been no long-term controlled trials involving atorvastatin, cerivastatin or fluvastatin.

Two trials involving fibrates have shown reductions in coronary heart disease events. Fibrates are not recommended as first-line lipid-lowering interventions because of concerns about adverse effects.

Box 8.8 Many people with established cardiovascular disease do not receive lipid lowering drugs[31]

The total cholesterol and lipid levels of more than 13 000 adults sampled from across England were measured. At least 25% had adverse lipid profiles. The proportion of adults taking lipid-lowering drugs was 2.2%. Less than one-third of patients with a history of coronary heart disease or stroke had received lipid-lowering drugs. Recently recommended targets for cholesterol concentrations were reached by only 1 in 10 people who were eligible for treatment.

Statins constitute the single most effective type of treatment for decreasing cholesterol levels and reducing cardiovascular risk. There is a depression of lipids following a myocardial infarction, which can last for an average of 6 weeks. It is therefore essential to measure the lipid profile 6 to 12 weeks after an acute myocardial infarction. This should be repeated in 6 to 12 weeks if it is below the threshold at the time of a coronary event.

The Scandinavian Simvastatin Survival Study (4S) randomised patients who had had a myocardial infarction, or who had angina with a positive exercise test. The intervention group received simvastatin, and the mean reduction in cholesterol levels after 5 years was 28%. The total mortality was reduced by 30%, and there was a 42% reduction in coronary heart disease deaths. The need for coronary artery surgery or angioplasty was also reduced. The Long-term Intervention with Pravastatin in Ischaemic Disease (LIPID) study confirmed and extended the findings of the 4S study in a larger series of patients.[29,30]

The data from some of the trials suggest that there may be little to be gained in primary prevention by lowering total serum cholesterol levels much below 5.0 mmol/L. Measurement of HDL/LDL ratios assume more importance in primary prevention.

The Cholesterol And Recurrent Events (CARE) study using pravastatin showed that even treating patients with average cholesterol levels (6.2 mmol/L per litre) produced a reduction in cholesterol levels, associated with decreases in CHD events and mortality. However, the overall mortality was not significantly reduced. Statins appear to provide benefits which are additional to those resulting from the use of other secondary prevention interventions, such as aspirin and beta-blocker drugs.

According to the Joint British Recommendations, the upper age limit for initiating lipid-lowering medication should be 75 years, and for primary prevention it should be 69 years.[2] The recommendation from the Scottish Intercollegiate Guidelines Network (SIGN) is that elderly patients on existing lipid-lowering therapy should not have their drugs stopped on account of their age.[13,14] However, until further evidence is obtained from trials, the evidence of benefit from using lipid-lowering drugs for primary prevention of coronary heart disease in men and women who are over 70 years of age remains uncertain.

The broad national cost implications for treating people who have at least a 30% risk threshold over 10 years would require 3.4% of the population aged 35–69 years to be treated for primary prevention, and 4.8% to be treated for secondary prevention, giving a total of 8.2% of the population. The total cost would be around £1 billion per annum for England. The costs include those of prescribing, screening and primary care services.

Box 8.9

It has been estimated that the cost of stains alone (for treating at or above the 30% risk level) is £200 000 for secondary prevention and £50 000 for primary prevention in a practice of 10 000 patients.[32]

An alternative approach to prioritising treatment with lipid-lowering therapy for the population, recommended in the SIGN guidelines, is to work with patients who are known to be at risk of at least 30%, and limit screening to individuals with:

- diabetes, including those with impaired glucose tolerance
- hypertension
- a family history of premature coronary heart disease (first-degree male relatives less than 55 years of age and female relatives less than 65 years)
- clinical signs of hyperlipidaemia
- smokers.[14]

ACE inhibitors[1]

Angiotensin-converting-enzyme (ACE) inhibitor drugs improve asymptomatic left ventricular dysfunction following myocardial infarction.

Patients with clinical evidence of heart failure following myocardial infarction showed a 27% reduction in the risk of death and a 19% reduction in vascular events following treatment with ACE inhibitors (*see* Chapter 6 for further details).

Anticoagulants[1]

There is some evidence that anticoagulant therapy reduces the risk of reinfarction and cerebrovascular events. However, the routine use of anticoagulants is not indicated, although anticoagulants are commonly used for large anterior myocardial infarcts and in patients with left ventricular aneurysms.

Anti-arrhythmic agents[1]

The evidence of the benefits of anti-arrhythmic agents following a myocardial infarction, in terms of a reduction in mortality, are not clear and further research is needed.

Aspirin[1,13,14]

The SIGN guidelines recommend that aspirin should be taken by all patients whose risk is at or above the 30% threshold. If the recommendation was to be applied to the lower 15% risk threshold of a coronary heart disease event occurring in the next 10 years, 60 people would need to be treated with aspirin for 5 years in order to avoid one coronary or stroke event. This benefit has to be balanced against the risk of provoking a gastrointestinal haemorrhage.

Hypertension

See Chapter 2 for a detailed consideration of hypertension.

Hormone replacement therapy (HRT)

The evidence for the effectiveness of HRT in preventing coronary heart disease is inconclusive.

Reality: the potential to improve secondary prevention

In a study of around 2000 patients in general practices in Scotland, researchers found considerable potential to increase secondary prevention in primary care. Only 63% of patients took aspirin, 32% took beta-blocker drugs and 40% of those with heart failure took angiotensin-converting-enzyme inhibitors. Hypertension management was consistent with current guidelines for 82% of patients but only 17% of patients had evidence-based management of hyperlipidaemia. Just over half (51%) took little or no exercise, 18% were smokers, 64% were overweight and 52% ate more fat than is recommended. For virtually all of the patients there was at least one aspect of their clinical management where care was suboptimal, and about 50% had suboptimal care for at least two aspects of their management. Similarly nearly all patients had at least one high-risk behaviour, and nearly two-thirds had at least two high-risk behaviours.[33]

The *number needed to treat* (NNT) is a useful measure of the effectiveness of medical interventions (*see* Table 8.2).

Investigations

The best lipid predictor of coronary heart disease is the ratio of total cholesterol to HDL cholesterol.

Measure triglyceride after a 12-hour fast in order to obtain an accurate value for baseline levels.

Exclude secondary causes of high lipids by checking the following:

- urea, creatinine and electrolytes
- urinanalysis
- fasting glucose
- liver function tests
- thyroid-stimulating hormone.

Table 8.2 Comparison of the treatment benefits from interventions to prevent cardiovascular events (adapted from Sivers, 1999[9])

Problem and therapy	Events prevented	Estimated number of patients who need to be treated for 5 years to prevent one event (NNT)
Medication for severe hypertension (diastolic blood pressure 115–129 mmHg)	Death, stroke or myocardial infarction	3
CABG for left main coronary artery disease	Death	6
Aspirin for transient ischaemic attack	Death or stroke	6
HMG-CoA reductase inhibitor (simvastatin) following myocardial infarction	Death, coronary event, CABG/PTCA or stroke	6
Warfarin for atrial fibrillation	Stroke	7
ACE inhibitor for left ventricular dysfunction following myocardial infarction	Cardiovascular death or hospitalisation for chronic heart failure	10
Aspirin following myocardial infarction	Cardiovascular death, stroke or myocardial infarction	12
Beta-blocker following myocardial infarction	Death	21
ACE inhibitor for left ventricular dysfunction	Cardiovascular death or hospitalisation for chronic heart failure	21
HMG-CoA reductase inhibitor for primary prevention	Death, coronary event, CABG/PTCA or stroke	26
Medication for mild hypertension (diastolic blood pressure 90–109 mmHg)	Death, stroke or myocardial infarction	141

Developing a coronary heart disease register

Just as for the priorities with regard to prevention and treatment listed in Box 8.2, set up your coronary heart disease register including those patients who have established vascular disease first of all. Then expand the disease register to include those at high-risk of developing a coronary heart disease event over a 10-year period. Include patients with diabetes or hypertension, and those of British Asian descent.

The following list indicates the minimum information about risk factors that should be included on the risk register:

- smoking status
- physical activity profile
- body mass index
- blood pressure
- serum cholesterol
- blood glucose or HbA_{1c} (for patients with diabetes).

A comprehensive guide to setting up an electronic disease register using coronary heart disease as an example is given elsewhere.[34]

A sample protocol for a nurse-led secondary prevention clinic can be found in Appendix 2.

Reflection exercises

Exercise 14

Invite the local cardiologist to the practice for an in-house educational session, and invite other practice teams to join you.

Discuss the ten last referral letters written to the hospital and the ten most recent letters written from the consultant to the practice. Could you have done more in the practice? Were the responding letters from the hospital staff appropriate? Do they need to learn more about the problems of general practice? Ask the consultant to review your practice protocol and discuss how to provide more seamless care for patients, shifting work and resources to primary care as far as possible.

Exercise 15

In a similar way to Exercise 14, invite the local community pharmacists, the community dietitian or staff from the local sports club to join you for an educational session.

Positively encourage them to contribute to reviewing a relevant practice protocol, or to take part in a general discussion of your learning needs as a practice in their specialty areas.

Exercise 16

Ask ten consecutive patients who smoke cigarettes who consult you to describe what risks they perceive they have of developing coronary heart disease, stroke or other consequences, such as cancers.

Do they have realistic perspectives? What educational indicators would be useful to inform them about the risks? Ask your local health education unit for help.

Exercise 17

Undertake an audit to determine the proportion of patients with diabetes who have a history of smoking recorded.

Randomly select 20 case-notes of patients with type 1 and type 2 diabetes for this exercise.

 (i) What proportion have had their smoking status recorded in the last year?
 (ii) How can this proportion be improved? Draw up an action plan and re-audit in 12 months' time.
(iii) Do you know which interventions for smoking cessation are most likely to be successful, and for which patients with diabetes they are warranted? How could you target these patients? Draw up an action plan for the interventions to be introduced in the monitoring system for patients with diabetes.

Exercise 18

Undertake a significant event audit around a serious adverse condition that has occurred recently (e.g. a patient under 50 years of age dying unexpectedly after having had a myocardial infarction 12 months previously).

Look at the circumstances leading up to the event. Discuss the case as a practice team, and consider whether you could have intervened more effectively at any time. Were the patient's risk factors well controlled? Were their smoking status, acceptable lipid levels and blood pressure readings and lifestyle habits recorded in the notes before and since the myocardial infarction one year ago? Could the management of this patient have been more effective?

Now that you have completed these interactive reflection exercises, transfer the information to the empty template of the personal development plan on pages 142–151 if you are working on your own learning plan, or to the practice personal and professional development plan on pages 165–172 if you are working on a practice team learning plan. Don't forget to keep the evidence of your learning in your personal portfolio.

References

1 Barton S (ed.) (2001) *Clinical Evidence. Issue 5.* BMJ Publishing Group, London.
2 Wood D, Durrington P, Poulter N *et al.* (1998) Joint British recommendations on prevention of coronary heart disease in clinical practice. *Heart.* **80 (Supplement 2)**: S1–29.
3 Iqbal Z, Chambers R and Woodmansey P (2001) *Implementing the National Service Framework for Coronary Heart Disease in Primary Care.* Radcliffe Medical Press, Oxford.
4 Machado F (1999) Prevention of coronary heart disease. *Update.* **9 April**: 605–11.
5 Moore A and McQuay H (eds) (2000) Better health through better lifestyle. *Bandolier.* **7**: 3–4.
6 Foord-Kelcey G (ed.) (2001) *Guidelines.* Medendium Group Publishing Ltd, Berkhamsted.
7 Office for National Statistics (2000) *Key Health Statistics from General Practice 1998.* Office for National Statistics, London.
8 Erens B, Primatesta P and Prior G (eds) (2001) *Health Survey for England: the health of minority ethnic groups '99.* Department of Health, London.
9 Sivers F (1999) *Evidence-Based Strategies for Secondary Prevention of Coronary Heart Disease* (2e). A and M Publishing, Guildford.
10 Chambers R, Stead J and Wakley G (2001) *Diabetes Matters in Primary Care.* Radcliffe Medical Press, Oxford.
11 Heart Outcomes Prevention Evaluation Study Investigators (2000) Effects of ramipril on cardiovascular and microvascular outcomes in people with diabetes mellitus: results of the HOPE and MICRO-HOPE substudy. *Lancet.* **355**: 253–9.
12 Turner RC, Mills H, Neil HA *et al.* (1998) Risk factors for coronary

heart disease in non-insulin-dependent diabetes mellitus: United Kingdom Prospective Diabetes Study. *BMJ.* **316**: 823–8.

13 Royal College of General Practitioners (Scotland), Scottish Heart and Arterial Disease Risk Prevention, and Scottish Intercollegiate Guidelines Network (2000) *The Heart Pack: coronary heart disease resource directory.* Royal College of General Practitioners, Edinburgh.

14 Scottish Intercollegiate Guidelines Network (1999) *Lipids and the Primary Prevention of Coronary Heart Disease.* SIGN Secretariat, Edinburgh.

15 Albert CM, Hennekens CH, O'Donnell CJ *et al.* (1998) Fish consumption and risk of sudden cardiac death. *JAMA.* **279**: 23–8.

16 National Heart Forum (1999) *Looking to the Future: making coronary heart disease an epidemic of the past.* The Stationery Office, London.

17 Office for National Statistics (2000) *Drug Use, Smoking and Drinking Among Teenagers in 1999.* Office for National Statistics, London.

18 Secretary of State for Health and Secretaries of State for Scotland, Wales and Northern Ireland (1998) *Smoking Kills: a White Paper on tobacco.* The Stationery Office, London.

19 Office for National Statistics (2000) *Living in Britain: results from the 1998 General Household Survey.* The Stationery Office, London.

20 Godfrey C, Raw M, Sutton M *et al.* (1993) *The Smoking Epidemic: a prescription for change.* Health Education Authority, London.

21 Action on Smoking and Health (ASH) *Basic Facts No 1. Smoking statistics, January 2000.* Action on Smoking and Health, London.

22 Peto R, Darby S, Deo H *et al.* (2000) Smoking, smoking cessation and lung cancer in the UK since 1950: combination of national statistics with two case–control studies. *BMJ.* **321**: 323–9.

23 NHS Executive (2000) *National Service Framework for Coronary Heart Disease.* Department of Health, London.

24 Fowler G (2000) Smoking cessation: a key role for primary care. *Update.* **May (Suppl.)**: 3–8.

25 Lancaster T, Stead L, Silagy C *et al.* for the Cochrane Tobacco Addiction Review Group (2000) Effectiveness of interventions to help people stop smoking: findings from the Cochrane Library. *BMJ.* **321**: 355–8.

26 Collier J (ed.) (2000) Bupropion to aid smoking cessation. *Drug Ther Bull.* **38**: 73–5.

27 Fowler G (2000) Helping smokers to stop: an evidence-based approach. *Practitioner.* **244**: 37–41.

28 Antiplatelet Triallists' Collaboration (1994) Collaborative overview of randomised trials of antiplatelet therapy. 1. Prevention of death, myocardial infarction and stroke by prolonged antiplatelet therapy in various categories of patients. *BMJ.* **308**: 81–106.

29 Scandinavian Simvastatin Survival Study Group (1995) Randomised trial of cholesterol lowering in 4444 patients with coronary heart disease: the Scandinavian Simvastatin Survival Study(4S). *Lancet.* **344**: 1383–9.

30 Long-term Intervention with Pravastatin in Ischaemic Disease (LIPID) Study Program (1998) Prevention of cardiovascular events and death with

pravastatin in patients with coronary heart disease and a broad range of initial cholesterol levels. *NEJM.* **339**: 1349–57.

31 Primatesta P and Poulter N (2000) Lipid concentrations and the use of lipid-lowering drugs: evidence from a national cross sectional survey. *BMJ.* **321**: 1322–5.

32 Campbell NC (1999) Edinburgh consensus conference on lipid lowering. *Trends Cardiol Vasc Dis.* **1**: 31–4.

33 Campbell NC, Thain J, George Deans H *et al.* (1998) Secondary prevention in coronary heart disease: baseline survey of provision in general practice. *BMJ.* **316**: 1430–44.

34 Gillies A, Ellis B and Lowe N (2002) *Building an Electronic Disease Register: getting the computers to work for you.* Radcliffe Medical Press, Oxford.

CHAPTER 9

Draw up and apply your personal development plan focusing on cardiovascular disease

You may want to focus on the clinical management of cardiovascular disease in general, or you may be interested in a specific aspect such as smoking cessation. A personal development plan (PDP) on either of these topics could form part of a practice personal and professional development plan (PPDP) (*see* Chapter 10). We have included a worked example of a personal development plan focused on smoking cessation on pages 130–141.

As we explained in the introduction, you may decide to allocate 50% of the time you intend to spend drawing up and applying a personal development plan in any one year to learning more about cardio-vascular disease. That would leave space in your learning plan for other important topics such as diabetes, mental healthcare or cancer – whatever is a priority for you, your practice team and your patient population. There will be some overlap between topics – you cannot consider a patient with stroke in isolation from their mental health and general well-being.

The worked example focusing on smoking cessation is compre-hensive, and you may not want to include so much detail in your own personal development plan. You might have a different approach and other educational activities, because your needs and circumstances are different to those of the example practitioners described here. You might move on to Chapter 10 and modify the worked example of a practice personal and professional development plan centred on coronary heart disease for your personal development plan.

Choose several methods to justify the topic that you have chosen or to identify your learning needs. Incorporate learning needs or baseline information from the reflection exercises at the end of each chapter, such as the clinical governance check-list from the material in Chapter 1 or the SWOT analysis in Chapter 2. Transfer the information about your learning needs from any of the reflection exercises at the end of the chapters that are relevant to you, and that you have completed, to the empty template of the personal development plan that follows on pages 142–151. The reflection exercises that you decide to select will depend on the focus of your personal development plan – as in the worked example here.

Draft your action learning plan. You might have already prepared this in one of the reflection exercises at the end of each chapter. Show it to someone else and ask for their views as to whether it is relevant, well balanced and achievable. Undertake your learning and demonstrate the subsequent improvements in your knowledge and practice.

Drawing up your personal development plan and carrying it out might take 10 to 20 hours depending on what topic you choose, the extent of preliminary needs assessment you carry out, how detailed your action learning plan is and the type of evaluation that you undertake.

Worked example of a personal development plan focusing on smoking cessation

What topic have you chosen?

Smoking cessation.

Who chose it?

You may have chosen the topic, but others in the practice may also have suggested that you take a lead on smoking cessation.

Why is the topic a priority?

(i) A personal or professional priority? You may not be familiar with the most up to date and effective approaches for helping patients to stop smoking. You might want to invest time and effort in health promotion to prevent ill health.

(ii) A practice priority? You will want to implement the most cost-

effective ways to deliver smoking cessation – and you may need to find out more.

(iii) A district priority? Smoking cessation is probably one of the priorities in your district's health improvement programme (HImP).

(iv) A national priority? Smoking cessation is a national priority, such as in the National Service Framework for Coronary Heart Disease in England.

Who will be included in your personal development plan?

You might involve the following:

- GP colleagues
- practice nurse
- health visitor
- community pharmacist
- receptionist to represent non-clinical staff.

(Although your personal development plan is about what *you* will learn, you should liaise with all of these people to agree a practice protocol and disseminate what you learn.)

What baseline information will you collect and how? How will you identify your learning needs?

You could ask the practice manager to find out details of any training in smoking cessation that is available.

Find out from the PCO or local health promotion department what is in the pipeline for the immediate and long-term future development of smoking cessation in your area. They may have a 'model' practice protocol on smoking cessation that you could individualise for your practice.

Run an audit on the practice computer to see how many patients are registered as current smokers and what other information you can extract about them (their risk profiles, etc.).

Undertake an audit to find out how many of the patients you have advised to stop smoking in the past have actually stopped. Look through the notes of the next 50 patients who consult you who are at risk of developing coronary heart disease or have established heart disease (e.g. those who have hypertension, diabetes, or a strong family history of heart disease). Sift out those who smoke cigarettes now or did so in the past. How many of them are still smoking? How many have stopped? For how many did you play a contributory part in helping them to stop? Ask both those that have and those that have not stopped smoking if they remember you giving them advice in the past, and whether they can remember what you said, or what you prescribed to help them quit, or what literature you gave them.

Read about smoking cessation in a compendium of evidence such as Barton S (ed.) (2001) *Clinical Evidence. Issue 5*. BMJ Publishing Group, London. How much did you know already, and how much have you got to learn?

Ask colleagues how well they think you perform with regard to changing patients' behaviour. They may have some insight into how good you are at motivating people to change.

What are the learning needs of the practice and how do they match your needs?

The reflection exercises earlier in the book should have already given you some information about your learning needs and those of the rest of the practice team. You may be focusing on smoking cessation, but you will also need to consider whether you have the necessary computer skills to set up templates for recording patients' smoking status and running audits, if you do not have those arranged already. If no one in the practice has these skills, you should include IT training in your personal development plan. If others do have these skills, ask them to teach you what you need to know in order to run the smoking cessation programme effectively.

Consider undertaking a SWOT analysis of either your own or the practice team's strengths, weaknesses, opportunities and threats with regard to smoking cessation, at a team meeting. In this way you will start to gauge the extent of the practice's learning and organisational needs, so that you develop a systematic approach to smoking cessation for all of your practice population. This SWOT exercise will help to gain their ownership of the initiative, too. For instance, it might reveal the following.

- *Strengths*: Enthusiasm. Willingness to learn (clinical evidence changes rapidly). Communication skills and inter-professional relationships to enable inter-disciplinary working. Organisational skills, teaching skills, and research skills to provide a resource for smoking cessation, once learned.
- *Opportunities*: The local pharmacist might have been trained in smoking cessation. A GP or practice nurse in a neighbouring practice may have been on an updating course and be enthusiastic to pass on his or her newly acquired knowledge. A course on managing changes in behaviour may be available.
- *Weaknesses and threats*: Deficiencies in your practice organisation with regard to record-keeping or availability of training. Other

commitments, antagonism or lack of support from others. Other staff being away on courses or involved with administrative tasks means that fewer people are available for routine work.

Is there any patient or public input to your personal development plan?

Do you have any patients' group that wants to be involved in helping to design how you might run the smoking cessation service so that it is convenient for patients? Ask them if they want the practice to set up a website (e.g. with information about staying healthy).

Hold a roadshow in the practice one evening or on a Saturday morning on the subject of stopping smoking. Advertise it widely. Interested patients attending will probably give you ideas about how the practice and the staff could improve the services, systems and procedures from a patient's perspective.

What mechanism(s) will you use to find out patients' views in a meaningful way, and not just the opinions of the most opinionated or compliant? You may need to think deeply about the reliability of any method, and how representative individual patients are of your whole practice population.

Aims of your personal development plan arising from the preliminary data-gathering exercise

1 To find out which interventions reduce cigarette smoking most effectively and apply those interventions in practice, resources permitting.
2 To learn how to motivate patients who smoke to stop smoking, and to apply that learning in practice.

How might you integrate the 14 components of clinical governance into your personal development plan focusing on smoking cessation?

As you work through this clinical governance check-list, identify what learning needs you have to match the service needs you identify, and shape your action learning plan accordingly. These needs might include learning more about time management, communication and negotiation to enable you to function more effectively within the team.

Establishing a learning culture: hold regular meetings (e.g. quarterly) on coronary heart disease. Share what you learn about smoking cessation with other practice team members, in order to transfer your new skills and information.

Managing resources and services: review whether you are targeting patients with established heart disease and diabetes appropriately and advising those who smoke to stop, and also how you fit in delegating or receiving others' referrals.

Establishing a research and development culture: search on the National Electronic Library for Medicine (*see* list of useful websites in Appendix 3) for evidence-based procedures and information to disseminate throughout the practice team, including the attached staff (e.g. for effective smoking cessation programmes).

Reliable and accurate data: enter data about smoking status once, consistently and correctly, be able to retrieve it for a variety of uses, and be able to compare the data with those of others. Lead your practice in deciding on and using consistent Read codes, or in transferring to SNOMED.

Evidence-based practice and policy: find out which interventions are most successful and the evidence for motivating people to change. Use *Bandolier* and York Centre for Reviews and Dissemination for updates (*see* list of useful websites in Appendix 3).

Confidentiality: ensure that you and others use passwords on the computer correctly and securely. Some smokers may be reluctant to be identified openly, concealing their smoking from their partner or place of work, etc., so develop a policy to cover the issues.

Health gain: helping people to stop smoking will have immense health gains for them if they are successful in quitting.

Coherent team: everyone needs to know how to refer patients who want to stop smoking, when to prescribe nicotine replacement treatments and other anti-smoking medication, and which patients are being targeted first.

Audit and evaluation: check your own and others' consistent entry of Read codes relating to smoking status and whether advice/help has been offered. Set up regularly repeating audits of recording.

Meaningful involvement of patients and the public: consider running a patient focus group to gather people's views. If you do not know how to run such a group and obtain meaningful information, weave that learning into your action plan, too.

Health promotion: target those at risk with specific reminders on the computer screen for particular groups of patients. If you do not know what constitutes 'at risk' or how to operate the computer in this way, include those elements in your learning plan as well. Learn about the range of techniques for smoking cessation.

Risk management: patients with diabetes who smoke are an 'at-risk' group with whom you could start. Agree your protocol with the practice team.

Accountability and performance: include your personal development plan and a record of the subsequent improvements that you make in your portfolio ready for revalidation or re-accreditation of your professional qualifications. You should be able to demonstrate how effective your learning has been. Review everyone who received smoking cessation help and advice 12 months later. How many of them are not smoking?

Core requirements: could you work out a better skill mix in your practice team to provide more cost-effective use of time spent on the care of patients with chronic diseases?

Action learning plan

Timetabled action.   Start date . . .

By 2 months: preliminary data gathered and colleagues working with you identified.
- Skills that are already present (your own, in practice, in the PCO, health promotion department in health authority, etc.).
- Equipment and systems that are available (your own, in the practice, in the PCO, outside in a training venue).
- Training that can be obtained (to match your needs).
- Training that could take place (in the practice, other practice(s), distance learning, some other local or distant venue).

- How it could be done (private study, individual or group; tutor led or cascade learning).

By 4 months: review current performance.
- Review the results of audits of how well you are able to motivate people to change their behaviour and stop smoking.
- Assess for how many people you know their smoking status. What proportion of the practice is this?
- Look at the opportunities arising from your SWOT analysis; look at the weaknesses you need to learn to rectify.
- Are your skills being utilised in the most effective way?
- Does the computer meet the specifications for the tasks you are required to perform now and those that you anticipate doing in the immediate future?

By 6 months: identify solutions and associated learning needs.
- Arrange the necessary training.
- Make a business plan for any associated equipment needs.
- Arrange cover for yourself and any other staff who are involved, to provide protected time for learning.
- Clarify who does what and when, in your practice protocol.
- Negotiate changes necessary at practice meeting(s).

By 12 months: make the changes and put your learning into practice.
- Implement the new systems or procedures.
- Obtain feedback from patients and other staff as to its impact.
- Iron out any difficulties.
- Identify any gaps in the provision.

Expected outcomes: an increasing proportion of patients (set exact target depending on your current baseline) with established heart disease, and those at risk of heart disease, have their smoking status recorded; smokers who receive 'stop smoking' advice actually quit; those who are ready to do so receive smoking cessation therapy; a practice protocol on smoking cessation is updated; all members of the practice team understand their roles and responsibilities – training needs fed into practice-based learning plan; you apply best practice in motivating patients to change their behaviour; reliable accurate data, easily entered and retrieved; relevant inter-disciplinary shared information.

How does your personal development plan tie in with your other strategic plans?

Smoking cessation is a priority for the PCO and the health improvement programme – so there should be local training programmes and resources to expedite learning and subsequent enhancement of service provision.

What additional resources will you require to execute your plan and from where do you hope to obtain them?

The PCO should be able to advise you on how to access local resources (*see* above).

How will you evaluate your personal development plan?

Set specific objectives before starting, and at timed intervals assess what progress you are making. Include some learning objectives and some targets of actual benefits for patients (e.g. number of patients giving up after you have helped them who have continued not to smoke at 6, 12 and 24 months). Also evaluate whether the type of learning activities you chose to pursue were the most appropriate for what you aimed to learn (e.g. small group teaching might be better than a lecture for a practical skill).

How will you know when you have achieved your objectives?

You can set up a system to follow up patients and measure the outcomes of smoking cessation therapy. Compare the figures before and after such intervention.

How will you disseminate the learning from your plan to the rest of the practice team and patients? How will you sustain your new-found knowledge or skills?

You can agree and monitor adherence to the practice protocol on smoking cessation and regular educational meetings on coronary heart disease for the practice team.

How will you handle new learning requirements as they crop up?

Record them in your portfolio, as practice meeting notes, etc.

Check out whether the topic you have chosen to learn is a priority and the way in which you plan to learn about it is appropriate

> **Your topic:** *smoking cessation.*

How have you identified your learning need(s)?

(a) PCO requirement	X	(e) Appraisal need ☐
(b) Practice business plan	X	(f) New to post ☐
(c) Legal mandatory requirement	☐	(g) Individual decision X
(d) Job requirement	☐	(h) Patient feedback ☐
		(i) Other ☐

Have you discussed or planned your learning needs with anyone else?

Yes ☒   No ☐   If so, who? *Practice team*

What are your learning need(s) and/or objective(s) in terms of the following?

Knowledge. What new information do you hope to gain to help you to do this?
Most effective interventions in smoking cessation.

Skills. What should you be able to do differently as a result of undertaking this learning in your development plan?
Be able to offer effective smoking cessation to the right people at the right time and be able to motivate them to change their smoking habit.

Behaviour/professional practice. How will this impact on the way in which you then subsequently do things?
I might be a more effective clinician. I might be a more effective tutor to other staff with regard to best practice in smoking cessation.

Details and date of desired development activity:
Details of courses, etc., could be included here.

Details of any previous training and/or experience that you have in this area/dates:

I attended a course on motivating obese people to lose weight – that would involve learning and skills which I can transfer to smoking cessation work.

What is your current performance in this area compared with the requirements of your job?

Need significant   ☒   Need some   ☐
development in this area   development in this area

Satisfactory in this area   ☐   Do well in this area   ☐

What is the level of job relevance that this area has to your role and responsibilities?

Has no relevance to job   ☐   Has some relevance   ☐

Relevant to job   ☐   Very relevant   ☒

Essential to job   ☐

Describe how the proposed education/training is relevant to your job:

I should know how to motivate people to adopt healthier behaviour and be able to demonstrate this skill by motivating and helping people who smoke to stop.

Do you need additional support in identifying a suitable development activity?

Yes   ☒   No   ☐

What do you need?

Practice manager is finding out about training opportunities.

Describe the differences or improvements for you, your practice, PCO and/or NHS trust as a result of undertaking this activity:

Help save some of the estimated £1.7 billion cost to the NHS from preventable deaths and illness secondary to smoking in the UK each year.

Assess the priority of your proposed educational/training activity:

Urgent ☐   High ☒   Medium ☐   Low ☐

Describe how the proposed activity will meet your learning needs rather than any other type of course or training on the topic:

A one-day course will allow me to focus on the topic and have time to learn practical skills.

If you had a free choice, would you want to learn this?   Yes/No

If No, why not? (please circle all that apply)

Waste of time
I have already done it
It is not relevant to my work or career goals
Other

If **Yes**, what reasons are most important to you? (put them in rank order)

To improve my performance   2
To increase my knowledge   1
To get promotion
I am just interested in it
To be better than my colleagues
To do a more interesting job   3
To enable me to be more confident   4
Because it will help me

Record of your learning about smoking cessation

You would write in the topic, date, length of time spent, etc., for each learning activity

	Activity 1 – learning how to motivate people	*Activity 2 – smoking cessation: effective interventions*	*Activity 3 – update IT skills*	*Activity 4 – writing the practice protocol*
In-house formal learning		Community pharmacist runs one-hour session on quitting smoking for all members of the practice team, and brings a range of nicotine replacement therapy	Spend an hour with computer operator in practice to update skills on recording smoking status, writing that into practice protocol; learning about running audits on computer	Write and present the protocol for identifying and referring smokers within the practice team
External courses	One-day course on motivating people to adopt healthier lifestyles	Learn about smoking cessation at same day course as for Activity 1		
Informal and personal	Reading and reflecting on articles in several months' issues of magazines; look for relevant papers in professional journals	Chat with others over coffee and lunch at day course and practice. Visit nearby practice to see how they do it		Obtain feedback informally from users of the protocol about how it is working
Qualifications and/or experience gained	Certificate of attendance at course			Keep the protocol in my portfolio, together with information about how it was produced

Reflection and planning exercise

Now complete your own personal development plan. It might be focused on a different topic to smoking cessation. It might be your personal perspective of the worked example of the practice personal and professional development plan focused on coronary heart disease, described in the next chapter. Alternatively, you might choose to tackle another aspect of coronary heart disease, such as secondary prevention – the choice is yours.

Photocopy the template of a personal development plan that is given on the following pages, or complete the version in the book. Choose a topic that meets your individual needs.

Template for your personal development plan

What topic have you chosen?

Who chose it?

Why is the topic a priority?

(i) A personal and professional priority?

(ii) A practice priority?

(iii) A district priority?

(iv) A national priority?

Who will be included in your personal development plan?
(Anyone other than you? Other GPs, employed staff, attached staff, others from outside the practice, patients?)

What baseline information will you collect and how? How will you identify your learning needs?
(How will you obtain this information and who will do it? Self-completion check-lists, discussion, appraisal, audit, patient feedback?)

What are the learning needs of the practice and how do they match your needs?

Is there any patient or public input to your personal development plan?

Aims of your personal development plan arising from the preliminary data-gathering exercise

How might you integrate the 14 components of clinical govern-ance into your personal development plan focusing on the topic of . . . . ?

As you work through this clinical governance check-list, identify what learning needs you have to match the service needs you identify, and shape your action learning plan accordingly. These needs might include learning more about time management, communication and negotiation to enable you to function more effectively within the team.

Establishing a learning culture:

Managing resources and services:

Establishing a research and development culture:

Reliable and accurate data:

Evidence-based practice and policy:

Confidentiality:

Health gain:

Coherent team:

Audit and evaluation:

Meaningful involvement of patients and the public:

Health promotion:

Risk management:

Accountability and performance:

Core requirements:

Action learning plan
(Include timetabled action and expected outcomes)

How does your personal development plan tie in with your other strategic plans?
(e.g. the practice's business or development plan, the primary care investment plan or the health improvement programme)

What additional resources will you require to execute your plan and from where do you hope to obtain them?
(Will you have to pay any course fees? Will you be able to organise any protected time for learning in working hours?)

How will you evaluate your personal development plan?

How will you know when you have achieved your objectives?
(How will you measure success?)

How will you disseminate the learning from your plan to the rest of the practice team and patients? How will you sustain your new-found knowledge or skills?

How will you handle new learning requirements as they crop up?

Check whether the topic you have chosen to learn is a priority and the way in which you plan to learn about it is appropriate

---

Your topic:

How have you identified your learning need(s)?

(a) PCO requirement ☐   (e) Appraisal need ☐

(b) Practice business plan ☐   (f) New to post ☐

(c) Legal mandatory requirement ☐   (g) Individual decision ☐

(d) Job requirement ☐   (h) Patient feedback ☐

             (i) Other ☐

Have you discussed or planned your learning needs with anyone else?

Yes ☐   No ☐   If yes, who?

. . . .

What are your learning need(s) and/or objective(s) in terms of the following?

Knowledge. What new information do you hope to gain to help you to do this?

. . . .

Skills. What should you be able to do differently as a result of undertaking this learning in your development plan?

. . . .

Behaviour/professional practice. How will this impact on the way in which you then subsequently do things?

. . . .

Details and date of desired development activity:

. . . .

Details of any previous training and/or experience you have in this area/dates:

. . . .

What is your current performance in this area compared with the requirements of your job?

Need significant development in this area	☐	Need some development in this area	☐
Satisfactory in this area	☐	Do well in this area	☐

What is the level of job relevance that this area has to your role and responsibilities?

Has no relevance to job	☐	Has some relevance	☐
Relevant to job	☐	Very relevant	☐
Essential to job	☐		

Describe how the proposed education/training is relevant to your job:

. . . .

Do you need additional support in identifying a suitable development activity?

Yes ☐   No ☐

What do you need?

. . . .

Describe the differences or improvements for you, your practice, PCO and/or NHS trust as a result of undertaking this activity:

. . . .

Assess the priority of your proposed educational/training activity:

Urgent ☐   High ☐   Medium ☐   Low ☐

Describe how the proposed activity will meet your learning needs rather than any other type of course or training on the topic:

. . . .

If you had a free choice, would you want to learn this?   Yes/No

If No, why not? (please circle all that apply)

Waste of time
I have already done it
It is not relevant to my work or career goals
Other

If Yes, what reasons are most important to you? (put them in rank order)

To improve my performance
To increase my knowledge
To get promotion
I am just interested in it
To be better than my colleagues
To do a more interesting job
To enable me to be more confident
Because it will help me

Record of your learning activities

Write in the topic, date, time spent, etc., for each learning activity

	Activity 1	Activity 2	Activity 3	Activity 4
In-house formal learning				
External courses				
Informal and personal				
Qualifications and/or experience gained				

CHAPTER 10

Draw up and apply your practice personal and professional development plan

The practice personal and professional development plan (PPDP) should cater for everyone who works in the practice. It will probably also include those attached to the practice. Clinical governance principles will balance the development needs of the population, the practice, the primary care organisation (PCO) *and* the individual personal development plans (PDPs) of your practice team.

You might want to start by asking everyone to identify their own learning needs, combining them with those of other people and then checking them against the practice business plan. You could start from the other direction, and develop a practice-based personal and professional development plan from your business plan and then identify everyone's individual learning needs within that. Whichever direction you start from, you must ensure that you integrate team members' individual needs with those of your practice and the needs and directives of the NHS.

Make your learning plan flexible. You may want to add something in later if circumstances suddenly change or an additional need becomes apparent – perhaps as the result of a complaint, the launch of a new drug or new requirements from the government, the PCO or the National Institute for Clinical Excellence (NICE).

Long-term locums (greater than six months, say), assistants, retained doctors and salaried GPs should all be included in the practice plan. Remember to include all those staff who work for the practice, however few their hours – you cannot manage without them or they would not be there!

Time is one of the resources that must be considered when drawing up your action plan. Adequate resources must be in place for your learning needs, and protected time must be built in.

Read the worked example through. It is not intended to be prescriptive, but merely a guide to the types of techniques you might use to identify your learning needs, define your objectives, undertake an assessment against the 14 components of clinical governance, and plan your action and evaluation. Then turn to the empty template that follows and start completing it by transferring the information that you have gathered from the range of reflection exercises at the end of each chapter.

Worked example of a practice personal and professional development plan focusing on coronary heart disease

Who chose the topic?
The practice team chose it as a result of undertaking a significant event audit after the unexpected death of Sid, a 45-year-old, from a myocardial infarction. The practice team agreed that coronary heart disease (CHD) should be a main topic in their practice personal and professional development plan, as there seemed to be so much that they needed to learn.

Why is the topic a priority?

(i) A practice priority? The practice team were horrified to find that they had never measured Sid's blood pressure or checked his cholesterol levels, despite the fact that he had a family history of heart disease, and had been seen three times in the 6 months preceding his death.

(ii) A district priority? The practice team were aware that CHD was a local priority in the district's health improvement programme. The district has higher morbidity and mortality rates for CHD than other comparable areas in the UK.

(iii) A national priority? CHD is a national priority, being the subject of a National Service Framework. The purpose of the NSF is to drive up quality and to tackle variations and inequalities in CHD care and services, both between different subgroups of the population and between different areas.

Who will be included in your practice personal and professional development plan?

You might include the following:

- GPs
- practice nurses
- practice manager
- receptionists
- district nurses
- community pharmacists
- health visitors
- public and patients.

Who will collect the baseline information and how?

The practice manager might collect background information about current performance, others' perspectives, options for standards and guidelines that they might adopt, available resources and sources of additional resources for the future.

Where possible, information could be requested from the primary care development manager of the PCO acting as a central resource of the information available within the PCO. The practice manager might organise receptionists and the practice secretary to help with the data collection.

The topic of CHD might include the management of angina, myocardial infarction, hypertension, and screening for and control of cholesterol levels.

You as a practice might collect information about the following:

- all recent practice-based initiatives – suggestions from patients/staff, minutes of practice meetings in the last 12 months which are relevant
- any recent audit of the extent to which aspirin is taken by those for whom it is clinically warranted with regard to their history of CHD
- the PCO's work-force plan describing how the practice's work-force numbers compare with those of their peers
- objectives of the PCO's primary care investment plan
- practice-based prescribing data on statins, hypertensive drugs and aspirin
- the health profile of the local community, including local morbidity and mortality rates from the health authority – compare any practice-specific data with district figures

- the health improvement programme and other relevant district health reports and strategies – how relevant do they seem to your circumstances? What can you learn from them to help you in your everyday work?
- any health needs survey that has already been undertaken by the local authority with regard to lifestyle habits
- information from local voluntary groups about how available they think services are in your practice, and their suggestions for improvements
- minutes of meetings of local community health forums – find out whether there is any mention of CHD matters
- district guidelines on referrals to the cardiology directorate – can you compare your referral patterns with those advised?
- published guidelines on managing cardiac conditions and hypertension – compare your practice protocols and see whether you can justify any variations.

What information will you obtain about individual learning wishes and needs?

The practice manager might talk to representatives of the practice team individually about the demands of their posts, priorities, roles and responsibilities as part of the appraisal. All members of the team could complete check-lists describing the following:

- their roles and responsibilities
- their own learning needs
- their comments on other team members' learning needs
- their ideas about what their standards of CHD care should be
- their personal aspirations and visions for the practice.

The practice manager could then collate this material and discuss it with the GP in the practice who leads on educational matters, and the practice nurse who is responsible for clinical governance. They might commission another case-note audit on hypertension, comparing your performance as a practice with that described in their preferred guidelines.

You might use any of the other methods for identifying and assessing learning needs as described throughout the reflection exercises in this book, such as observing how other practices do it (could one of the practice nurses or receptionists make an exchange visit with a member of staff in another practice?).

What are the learning needs of the practice and how do they match the needs of the individual?

The practice might prioritise learning according to the requirements of the standards in the National Service Framework on Coronary Heart Disease for England, relevant to the primary care setting.

Any individual staff members who put themselves forward to learn more about any of these particular topics are likely to find that their learning can be prioritised if the practice is weak in that area – such as how to undertake an intervention or motivate patients to do so, how to apply audit in practice, introducing more effective management of CHD as a whole or of one of the conditions that falls under the umbrella of CHD. This might involve a practice nurse learning more about smoking cessation, or a GP attending an update on the prescribing of statins, or a secretary learning more about efficient ways of managing practice disease registers.

Is there any patient or public input to your plan?

You might target patients who do not attend or who do not comply with recommended treatment and find out why this is so by asking them directly.

You might set up a patient panel within your adult practice population. Randomly select 30 patients from your practice list, write to them and invite them to participate – either in occasional face-to-face meetings or in a quarterly postal survey. Ask them whether you have got your services right – whether they are convenient, accessible and appropriate. Pose questions that are relevant to CHD.

How will you prioritise everyone's needs in a fair and open way?

A practice meeting might be devoted to the following:

- discussing and sorting all of the information about performance
- the team members' views about possible improvements
- the importance of the learning needs that have been identified
- the priorities for the practice
- considering the impact of the PCO's plans
- the practice circumstances, aspirations and plans for changes to services.

A 'Hanging Committee' consisting of a GP, a nurse and the practice manager could then be convened to prioritise the educational plan for the practice focused on coronary heart disease.

Aims of the practice personal and professional development plan arising from the preliminary data-gathering exercise:

To develop a learning programme that underpins the achievement of the following milestones:

- incorporating evidence-based interventions for the secondary prevention of CHD
- achieving the various milestones within the standards of the National Service Framework for Coronary Heart Disease for England, such as maintaining good records
- establishing, maintaining and using a register of patients with CHD
- undertaking regular and systematic clinical audit
- adhering to a locally agreed protocol on assessment, treatment and follow-up of CHD patients.

How might you integrate the 14 components of clinical governance into your practice personal and professional development plan focusing on CHD?

As you work through this clinical governance check-list, identify what learning needs you have to match the service needs you have identified, and shape your action learning plan accordingly. These needs might include learning more about time management, motivation, communication and negotiation to enable you to function more effectively as a team.

Establishing a learning culture: review the application of the practice protocol for responding to a myocardial infarction. This should involve all members of the practice staff in multidisciplinary learning about their roles and responsibilities – from the receptionist who recognises the urgency and arranges ambulance transport, to the GP who decides whether he or she can reach the patient before the ambulance to provide aspirin, pain relief and a defibrillator, and to ensure that all staff are up to date with cardiopulmonary resuscitation training.

Managing resources and services: equipment (e.g. sphygmomanometers, defibrillator, emergency bag with relevant drugs) should be regularly checked and in good order. Secondary prevention with statins should be a cost-effective option in that you should ultimately save on the costs of secondary care cardiac services and save human lives.

Establishing a research and development culture: investigate whether there are any differences in the levels of treatment and investigation between men and women or different ethnic groups that are not accounted for by the severity of their conditions.

Reliable and accurate data: establish a reliable way of identifying patients with CHD and an accurate way of classifying their condition and cataloguing their tests so that you can offer patients the most effective preventive treatment and monitor their response.

Evidence-based practice and policy: cite evidence for prescribing statins if your drug budget is inflated, according to recommended guidelines for best practice.

Confidentiality: patients should give informed permission before being subjected to any activities that fall outside usual NHS practice (e.g. taking part in any research study into the treatment or management of CHD, or being videotaped for educational purposes).

Health gain: CHD is one condition for which there is a great deal of evidence about how many lives are saved by using effective treatments. This is often described as the number needed to treat (NNT) with a specific intervention giving a beneficial health gain.

Coherent team: good teamwork is essential for managing patients with CHD, as many different disciplines and both clinical and non-clinical staff all play a part in prevention and the various stages of acute and chronic treatment.

Audit and evaluation: audit whether prescribing is rational and consistent, whether patients comply with treatment and advice, numbers of smokers, etc.

Meaningful involvement of patients and the public: hold an open evening in the practice on the theme of CHD, at which you not only give patients as a whole more information about preventing CHD and effective management, but you also invite patient feedback about your services. Act on this feedback in order to make it 'meaningful', and make changes to your practice's systems and services as appropriate.

Health promotion: smoking cessation and reductions in salt intake and body weight all decrease the risks of CHD.

Risk management: reduce the risks of individuals with CHD by more effective prevention and management, or reduce the risks of a mistake or omission in a practice service by introducing tighter procedures or better monitoring systems.

Accountability and performance: with the good teamwork that involves a wide range of staff from different disciplines all playing their part comes the need for clear lines of accountability.

Core requirements: organise the skill mix within the practice team so that the additional task of making improvements to cardio-vascular care and services is done and the routine work of the practice is covered.

Action learning plan

Agree who is involved/setting: as for staff set out previously – specify names, posts, timetabled action and start date.

By 3 months: preliminary data gathering and collation of baseline of providers.
- Are there practice protocols for the management of the various components of CHD – angina, myocardial infarction, secondary prevention, hypertension, screening for and control of cholesterol levels, smoking cessation, etc?
- Numbers of staff; map expertise; list other providers.
- Referral patterns for CHD conditions – acute admissions and routine.
- Information about the characteristics of those recorded on the practice computer as having CHD, including breakdown by gender, age and coexisting conditions (e.g. diabetes).
- Any relevant local and national priorities, and any additional associated resources for which you might apply.
- Staff report problems that limit the accessing of services, observed problems, views and suggestions.

By 5 months: review current performance.
- Practice manager reviews operation of services and closeness of working relationships with those in other organisations and sectors that have an interest in, or responsibility for, CHD (e.g. cardiac rehabilitation).
- Clinical lead reviews the extent of knowledge and skills of the practice team with regard to routine care of all aspects of CHD.
- Audit actual performance vs. pre-agreed criteria (e.g. with regard to referrals, health promotion, management, investigation and compliance).
- Compare performance with any or several of the 14 components of clinical governance (e.g. clinical risk management would be very relevant).

By 6 months: identify solutions and associated training needs.
- Set up new systems for access to services appropriate to people's needs.
- Give the practice team in-house training in dealing with patients with various conditions grouped under the umbrella of CHD.
- Revise the practice protocol on provision of routine and emergency management in order to address identified gaps in care, having undertaken a search for other evidence-based protocols. Agree roles and responsibilities as a team for delivering care and services according to the protocol, and arrange for certain staff to attend external courses. Arrange for the practice nurse or a GP to provide some in-house training to other GPs and nurses, the community pharmacist or others from outside organisations with whom the practice is liaising about the issues.

By 12 months: make changes.
- Clinicians adhere to practice protocol – as shown by repeat audits.
- Change times and locations of services to ones that are more appropriate for patients who have CHD or who are being screened for risk factors. Organise training to anticipate new requirements (e.g. train the practice nurse in detecting and controlling risks of CHD).

Expected outcomes: more effective prevention of CHD in general; better compliance with treatment and healthy lifestyle advice; revised practice protocols for the management of hypertension and control of hyperlipidaemia; ultimately lives saved.

How does your practice personal and professional development plan tie in with your other strategic plans?

CHD might be a key item in the annual priority-setting exercise for the practice business plan. The extent of education and development needed would be revealed by the preliminary needs assessment, the high CHD mortality and morbidity rates of the local population, and the realisation that the practice should invest in two new defibrillators (for the doctor on call and for the practice treatment room).

The practice personal and professional development plan that focuses on CHD will tie in with the National Service Framework on coronary heart disease and subsidiary local initiatives.

What additional resources will you require to execute your plan and from where do you hope to obtain them?

The practice might pay for the course fees of any member of staff who undertakes training that fulfils a priority need of the practice.

You may be able to justify an application to your PCO for additional resources based on your preliminary learning and health needs assessments, tapping into the district or national strategic priorities.

If a member of staff is undertaking the training on behalf of the practice you should try to arrange for the training to be undertaken in paid time. Any learning that is cascaded to other members of the practice team as part of the practice personal and professional development plan should also be undertaken in paid time and during working hours whenever possible.

How will you evaluate your practice personal and professional development plan?

The specific evaluation activities will depend on the aims and content of the learning plan. The practice might re-audit their management of hypertension, hyperlipidaemia and post-myocardial infarction one year after embarking on the plan.

A SWOT analysis undertaken as part of the preliminary needs assessment will lend itself to review once the learning plan is in place or completed, in order to note the changes that have occurred and the extent to which 'weaknesses' have been redressed and 'threats' minimised.

Other techniques that were described with regard to assessing and identifying learning needs in the first section of the book might be used for evaluation, too, such as observation of practice, review of achievements during subsequent educational or job appraisals, or a repeat computer search to check developments with the CHD register.

How will you know when you have achieved your objectives?

Usually this will be by comparing the outcomes of your programme with the baseline data. You should undertake your evaluation so as to be able to demonstrate the extent to which you have met the milestones you set when you constructed your learning plan.

How will you disseminate the learning from your plan and sustain the developments and new-found knowledge or skills?

A member of the practice might attend the local community forum where health matters and community safety are always on the agenda – to give and receive information relating to CHD among other health issues.

A practice 'away-day' would provide a good opportunity to share learning and plan how to reorganise the practice team to provide more effective care for patients with CHD. Training could then be arranged for those who require additional knowledge and skills to fulfil their new roles and responsibilities with regard to the intended changes in methods of working.

How will you handle new learning requirements as they crop up?

The practice manager might run audits at intervals and feed the results back to a practice meeting mid-way through the time period of the practice personal and professional development plan, when there is time to revise the activities.

Record of practice team learning about cardiovascular disease

You would add the date, length of time spent etc., for each learning activity

	Activity 1 – establishing and maintaining a disease register for CHD	Activity 2 – reviewing practice protocols	Activity 3 – targeting appropriate secondary interventions	Activity 4 – learning about rehabilitation
In-house formal learning	Practice development manager from PCO spends 30 minutes of a practice meeting advising on new systems, after which practice agree who will do what, facilitated by practice manager	Four weekly sessions considering hypertension, angina, myocardial infarction, and screening for and controlling risks of CHD, attended by GPs, nurses and practice managers. Held with six local practices and facilitated by PCO clinical governance lead		Set up a local half-day learning session, inviting all relevant professions allied to medicine (PAMs) to set up displays of what rehabilitation they can offer. All members of the practice teams, district nurses and PAMs can tour the stations or stands to find out what is available
External courses			Practice nurse and GP attend two-day residential course on topic, and afterwards they run a small group session for others in the practice	
Informal and personal	GPs and practice nurse read about 'how to do it' in medical weekly newspaper, and then discuss how the suggested method would work in your practice over coffee. Later feed into in-house training (see above)	Chatting together during in-house weekly sessions (see above) gives plenty of food for thought. Many participants at sessions do further reading in their own time to prepare for the next session		Discuss what the practice team learned over tea/coffee and how to utilise the available resources more consistently for patients recovering from heart attacks and strokes
Qualifications and/or experience gained	Record your learning – and subsequent changes in practice	Keep a record of your part in drawing up practice protocols	GP and nurse put course materials in their own portfolios	Record your learning and how you will use it

Reflection and planning exercise

Now build up and complete your practice personal and professional development plan. It might be focused on another topic as well as tackling coronary heart disease. Then you can mesh the personal development plans of everyone else in the practice team.

Photocopy the template of a practice personal and professional development plan that is given on the following pages, or complete the version in the book. Choose a topic that meets your individual practice needs.

The practice manager or a GP with responsibility for education might take a lead on this exercise. They will have to lead and motivate the team, anticipate skill needs for any planned changes in the way in which you will be delivering coronary heart disease care and services, and organise appropriate education and training in good time.

- Ensure good communications within the practice about the learning plan.
- Organise regular staff meetings and separate educational meetings with team members and GPs. Invite attached staff to attend as appropriate.
- Be prepared to listen to staff and to seek their involvement in changes.
- Agree protocols in clinical and organisational work practices and adhere to them.
- Monitor performance regularly and appraise staff. Move away from a blame culture, and use mistakes as learning opportunities (try anyway!).

Template for your practice personal and professional development plan

What topic have you chosen?

Who chose it?

Why is the topic a priority?

(i) A personal and professional priority?

(ii) A practice priority?

(iii) A district priority?

(iv) A national priority?

Who will be included in your practice personal and professional development plan?
(GPs, employed and attached staff, others from outside the practice, patients?)

What baseline information will you collect and how?

How will you identify your learning needs? How will you obtain this information and who will do it?
(Self-completion check-lists, discussion, appraisal, audit, patient feedback?)

What are the learning needs of the practice and how do they match your needs?

Is there any patient or public input to your practice personal and professional development plan?

Aims of your practice personal and professional development plan arising from the preliminary data-gathering exercise
(e.g. reflection exercises throughout the book)

How might you integrate the 14 components of clinical governance into your personal development plan focusing on the topic of ....?

As you work through this clinical governance check-list, identify what learning needs practice team members have to match the service needs you identify, and shape your action learning plan accordingly. These needs might include learning more about time management, communication and negotiation to enable you to function more effectively within the team.

Establishing a learning culture:

Managing resources and services:

Establishing a research and development culture:

Reliable and accurate data:

Evidence-based practice and policy:

Confidentiality:

Health gain:

Coherent team:

Audit and evaluation:

Meaningful involvement of patients and the public:

Health promotion:

Risk management:

Accountability and performance:

Core requirements:

Action learning plan
(Include timetabled action and expected outcomes)

How does your practice personal and professional development plan tie in with your other strategic plans?
(e.g. the practice's business or development plan, the primary care investment plan or the health improvement programme)

What additional resources will you require to execute your plan and from where do you hope to obtain them?
(Will you have to pay any course fees? Will you be able to organise any protected time for learning in working hours?)

How will you evaluate your practice personal and professional development plan?

How will you know when you have achieved your objectives?
(How will you measure success?)

How will you disseminate the learning from your plan to the rest of the practice team and patients? How will you sustain your new-found knowledge or skills?

How will you handle new learning requirements as they crop up?

Record of your learning activities

Write in the topic, date, time spent, etc., for each type of learning activity

	Activity 1	Activity 2	Activity 3	Activity 4
In-house formal learning				
External courses				
Informal and personal				
Qualifications and/or experience gained				

Read codes for coronary heart disease

Developed by East Staffordshire Primary Care Group and Queens Hospital, Burton.

Diagnosis

G3 . . .	Ischaemic heart disease
G30 . .	Acute myocardial infarction
G33 . .	Angina

Coronary artery procedures

7928 .	Percutaneous transluminal coronary angioplasty
792 . .	Coronary artery bypass graft

Cardiac conditions

G5730	Atrial fibrillation
G58 . .	Heart failure
G6 . . .	Cerebrovascular disease
G65 . .	Transient cerebral ischaemia
G73 . .	Peripheral vascular disease: artery/arteriole and capillary disease

Investigations

3213 .	Exercise stress test
32130	Normal
32131	Abnormal
321 . .	Resting ECG
Normal Y/N	
Abnormal Y/N	

Echocardiogram

58530	Normal
58531	Abnormal

Risk factors

137 . .	Smoking status
1371 .	Never smoked
137S .	Ex-smoker
137R .	Current smoker
6791 .	Advice given
C10 . .	Diabetes mellitus
C108 .	Insulin-dependent diabetes
C109 .	Non-insulin-dependent diabetes
14A2 .	Hypertension
2469 .	Systolic blood pressure
246A .	Diastolic blood pressure
44P . .	Serum cholesterol
44P1 .	Normal
44P2 .	Raised
22K . .	BMI
22K4	BMI 25–29 (overweight)
22K5	BMI ≥ 30 (obese)
138 . .	Exercise
1385 .	Very active
1384 .	Moderate
1383 .	Light
1382 .	Inactive
136 . .	Alcohol
1361 .	Teetotaller
1364 .	Moderate drinker (3–6 units per day)
1365 .	Heavy drinker (7–9 units per day)
1366 .	Very heavy drinker (> 9 units per day)

Family history

Diagnosed coronary heart disease

12C2 .	Immediate family
Mother/sister	< 65 years Y/N
Father/brother	< 60 years Y/N

Hypertension
12C1 .   Immediate family
Mother/sister   < 65 years   Y/N
Father/brother   < 60 years   Y/N

Cerebrovascular accident/stroke/transient ischaemic attack
12C4 .   Immediate family
Mother/sister   < 65 years   Y/N
Father/brother   < 60 years   Y/N

Symptom/angina control

662K0	Stable	
662K1	Poor	
662K2	Improving	} Picking list within template
662K3	Deteriorating	
662Kz	NOS*	

Secondary prevention therapy

Health education
6791 .   Advice on smoking
6792 .   Advice on alcohol consumption
6798 .   Advice on exercise
6799 .   Advice on diet

8B28 .   Lipid-lowering therapy

8B63 .   Aspirin – includes over the counter
8124 .   Aspirin contraindication

8B69 .   Beta-blocker prophylaxis
8162 .   Beta-blocker not indicated
8B6B .   ACE-inhibitor prophylaxis

ZV579   Cardiac rehabilitation

662N .   Recall

* NOS = not otherwise specified

Detailed example of a protocol for a nurse-led clinic for the secondary prevention of cardiovascular disease

(Modified and then reproduced with the permission of North Stoke Primary Care Trust.)

The following working example has been developed by a primary care trust in the West Midlands. It describes the clinic protocol and the proposed audit parameters.

Aims

This protocol aims to achieve the NSF target *to identify all patients with established cardiovascular disease and offer them comprehensive advice and appropriate treatment to reduce their risks.*

Stage 1 – identification

Patients with established arterial disease are the first priority.

A register of all patients with cardiovascular disease will be maintained for the following:

- ischaemic heart disease
- myocardial infarction

- angina
- coronary artery bypass graft or angioplasty
- arteriosclerosis and peripheral vascular disease.

A separate register will include patients with cerebrovascular disease, stroke and transient cerebral ischaemia. The computer also maintains a register of patients with hypertension.

These registers will be maintained by:

- summarising all records, including new records entering the practice
- entering diagnoses from hospital discharge and out-patient reports
- entries made at the time of diagnosis in surgery.

Stage 2 – assessment

All patients with arterial disease should have a full assessment.

- Blood pressure should be measured in the sitting position, after the patient has been resting for 5 minutes, using an appropriate cuff size. Diastolic pressure should be phase 5, and blood pressure should be read to the nearest 2 mmHg. *It should be taken twice at each visit.*
- Blood tests for urea and electrolytes (U & Es), full blood count, total and HDL cholesterol, glucose and liver function tests should be performed annually.
- Urinalysis – dipstick testing should be performed annually.

Transfer any newly diagnosed hypertensives on to the hypertension protocol.

- Blood lipids – total and HDL cholesterol will be measured fasting ideally, or non-fasting followed by fasting if raised.

If the total cholesterol concentration is <5 mmol/L, reassure the patient. If the total cholesterol concentration is ≥ 5 mmol/L, refer the patient back to the doctor for treatment.

Stage 3 – assessment of risk

All patients with evidence of arterial disease, including previous myocardial infarct, angina, peripheral artery disease, or cerebrovascular disease are at high-risk of subsequent events and should receive advice and treatment to reduce that risk.

Use the standard ischaemic heart disease template on your practice computer.

Stage 4 – lifestyle advice

All patients will be offered lifestyle advice as appropriate. Patients will be advised to reduce their cardiovascular risk by:

- stopping smoking
- eating a prudent diet, following the Committee on Medical Aspects of Food Policy (COMA) recommendations, low in saturated fat, supplemented with polyunsaturated fats and fish oils, and high in fresh fruit and vegetables
- being moderately physically active
- keeping alcohol consumption below the recommended limits of up to 3–4 units per day for men and up to 2–3 units per day for women.

The lifestyle advice will follow a patient-centred approach with four stages as follows:

1 eliciting the patient's views, beliefs and readiness to change
2 explaining the nature of and reasons for advice
3 negotiating and agreeing goals
4 supporting the patient in achieving and maintaining change, and reinforcing this with appropriate health promotion materials.

Stage 5 – management of risk factors

Smokers

Patients who actively want to stop smoking should be offered detailed advice, including nicotine replacement therapy (or bupropion if appropriate) and follow-up.

Aspirin

All patients with arterial disease should be advised to take 75 mg aspirin daily unless this is contraindicated. If it is contraindicated, refer the patient to their GP for advice.

Lifestyle advice

All patients with CHD should receive appropriate lifestyle advice with particular emphasis on weight reduction, moderate alcohol intake and physical activity to reduce blood pressure, and smoking cessation and diet to reduce CHD risk.

Follow-up

This should take place monthly until controlled or maximal therapy is established, and then 6-monthly. All patients should have a full reassessment every 5 years. Patients on diuretics or ACE inhibitors should have their urine and electrolytes measured annually.

Indications for referral to GP

These include the following.

- New symptoms (e.g. chest pain, increasing shortness of breath, claudication). Urgency will depend on the nature of the symptoms.
- Poor control of blood pressure or lipids. Check adherence to treatment and either repeat the measurement or refer the patient back, depending on the levels.
- Side-effects, anxiety or difficulty in adhering to medication. Arrange a routine appointment as appropriate.

Audit requirements of this protocol

The performance of the programme will be reviewed annually. This will include the following.

1 Completeness of the arterial disease, cerebrovascular disease and hypertension registers by comparison with published prevalence, and by cross-checks with diagnostic codes and prescribing. Number identified, comparison of percentage figures with others' prevalence data, such as age–gender distribution of coronary vascular diseases in a typical practice of 10 000 patients (*see* Iqbal Z, Chambers R and Woodmansey P (2001) *Implementing the National Service*

Framework for Coronary Heart Disease in Primary Care. Radcliffe
Medical Press, Oxford).

2 Recording of risk factors and levels of control in patients on the
   registers, including smoking habits, blood pressure, BMI, physical
   activity and cholesterol. General recording of Read codes and
   consistency, etc.

3 Clinic attendance, and the number of patients on the register not
   seen for more than 12 months. Search on attendance at clinic per
   clinic code.

4 Prescribing rates for aspirin and lipid-lowering drugs for patients on
   the registers.

5 Screening – the proportions of the population, categorised by sex and
   10-year age groups, with recordings of:

   • blood pressure
   • smoking habits
   • significant family history.

Sources of information and support: organisations, websites, self-help groups and training programmes

Evidence-based resources

Agency for Health Care Policy and Research (AHCPR)	http://www.guideline.gov
Bandolier	http://ebandolier.com and http://www.jr2.ox.ac.uk/Bandolier/ band9/b9–1.html

The *Bandolier* site summarises issues relating to smoking cessation in a simple text format.

Canadian Medical Association	http://www.cma.ca/cpgs/
Cochrane Collaboration	http://www.cochrane.org and http://hiru.mcmaster.ca/cochrane

The Cochrane Review provides an index of general resources on smoking.

***Effective Health Care Bulletin* on cardiac rehabilitation from Centre for the Disseminations of Reviews**	http://www.york.ac.uk/inst/crd/ ehcb.htm
*e*Guidelines	http://www.eguidelines.co.uk
Guideline Project	http://www.ihs.ox.ac.uk/library/ librarylinks.htm#
Health Evidence Bulletins Wales	http://hebw.uwcm.ac.uk/
HoN (Health on the Net)	http://www.hon.ch
Medline	http://www.omni.ac.uk/medline
New Zealand Guidelines Group	http://www.nzgg.org.nz/
NLM Health Services/Technology Assessment	http://www.nlm.nih.gov

North of England Evidence-Based
Guidelines
OMNI (Organising Medical
Networked Information)
Pathways to the NSF

PRODIGY
Scottish Intercollegiate Guidelines
Network (SIGN)
St George's Health Care Evaluation
Unit
UK Health Centre

WISDOM Centre

http://www.ncl.ac.uk/~ncenthsr/
publicn/publicn.htm
http://www.omni.ac.uk

http://www.nsfpathways.co.uk/
nsf_pathways_homepage.html
http://www.prodigy.nhs.uk
http://www.sign.ac.uk

http://www.sghms.ac.uk/depts/phs/
hceu/nhsguide.htm
http://www.healthcentre.org.uk/hc/
pages/guidegeneral.htm
http://www.wisdomnet.co.uk

Official documents

http://www.official-documents.co.uk/document/doh/tobacco/contents.htm

A quick route to the many official documents, including a list of hyperlinks
papers behind the national strategy.

US sites

http://www.stop-smoking-secrets.com/
http://www.surgeongeneral.gov/tobacco/
http://www.cdc.gov/tobacco/

Relevant organisations

Action Heart, Wellesley House, 117 Wellington Road, Dudley DY1 1UB.
Tel: 01384 230222.

British Association for Nursing in Cardiac Care (BANCC), c/o British Cardiac
Society, 9 Fitzroy Square, London WIT 5HW. For all nurses, midwives and
health visitors who are interested in coronary heart disease.

British Heart Foundation, 14 Fitzharding Street, London W1H 4DH.
Tel: 0207 935 0185. Fax: 0207 486 1273. Website: www.bhf.org.uk

British Hyperlipidaemia Association, c/o David Middleton Communications,
Environmental Business Centre, B & IC, Aston Science Park, Birmingham
B7 4BJ. Tel: 0121 693 8338. Fax: 0121 693 8448. Email: ebc@dircon.co.uk

British Hypertension Society, Information Service, 127 High Street, Teddington, Middlesex TW11 8HH. Tel: 0208 977 0012. Fax: 0208 977 0055.

Diabetes UK, 7th Floor, Elizabeth House, 22 Suffolk Street, Queensway, Birmingham B1 1LS. Tel: 0121 643 5488. Fax: 0121 633 4399. Email: bda@dial.pipex.com

Family Heart Association, PO Box 303, Maidenhead SL6 9UX. Tel: 01628 628638.

Health Education Board of Scotland (HEBS), Website: http://www.hebs.scot.nhs.uk

The Scottish equivalent of the Health Development Agency site contains many graphics and animations.

National Patients' Access Team, 2A New Walk, Leicester LEI 6TF. Tel: 0116 254 8126. Fax 0116 255 2147.

PRIMIS (Primary Care Information Services), 14th Floor, Tower Building, University Park, University of Nottingham, Nottingham NG7 2RD. Tel: 0115 846 6420.

Guidelines and instructions on implementing a data quality improvement scheme for coronary heart disease can be downloaded free from the following websites:

http://www.primis.nhs.uk
http://www.primis.nottingham.ac.uk/
http://www.nottingham.ac.uk/chdgp/guidelin.htm
http://www.nottingham.ac.uk/chdgp/handbook.htm

Scottish Heart and Arterial Risk Prevention (SHARP) Group, Department of Medicine, Ninewells Hospital and Medical School, Dundee DD1 9SY. Tel: 01382 660111. Fax: 01382 660675. Email: srmcewan@ninewells.dundee.ac.uk

Stroke Association, Northampton Resource Centre, 61–69 Derngate, Northampton NN1 1HD.

Tobacco Campaign Helpline Service, Tel: 0800 1690169.

Walking the Way to Health Initiative (WHI)
Contact:
Countryside Agency. Tel: 01242 533258
or Countryside Council for Wales. Tel: 01248 385686. Website: www.whi.org.uk

This initiative provides grants to run projects aimed at improving people's health through walking, and offers face-to-face advice and support. Grants are mainly available for urban areas where people's health is poor, and the emphasis is on ethnic minority communities.

Coronary heart disease websites

UK

ASH – Action on Smoking and Health   http://www.ash.org.uk

BBC Education Heart Special   http://www.bbc.co.uk/education/
health/heart/

Blood Pressure Association   http://www.bpassoc.org.uk
British Cardiac Patients Association   http://www.cardiac-bcpa.co.uk/
index.html

British Cardiac Society   http://www.bcs.com/
British Heart Foundation (BHF)   http://www.bhf.org.uk/
**British Heart Foundation Statistics
    Database**   http://www.dphpc.ox.ac.uk/bhfhprg/
stats/index.html
British Hypertension Society   http://www.hyp.ac.uk/bhs/
Cardiac Rehabilitation   http://
www.cardiacrehabilitation.org.uk/

Cardiomyopathy Association   http://www.cardiomyopathy.org/
homepage.htm

Chest, Heart and Stroke, Scotland   http://www.chss.org.uk/
Children's Heart Federation   http://www.childrens-heart-
fed.org.uk/

Coronary Prevention Group   http://www.healthnet.org.uk/new/
cpg/index.htm

Giving Up Smoking   http://www.givingupsmoking.co.uk/
This is another national site, backed by the NHS, designed for those trying to
give up smoking, rather than for professionals.
**GUCH (Grown Up Congenital Heart
    Patients Association)**   http://www.guch.demon.co.uk/
index.htm
Heart (Journal)   http://heart.bmjjournals.com/
Heart Link Support Group   http://www.heartlink.org.uk/
National Electronic Library for Stroke   http://www.nhsia.nhs.uk/nelh/
vbranchlibs/stroke.asp

National Heart Forum   http://www.heartforum.org.uk/
Quit Smoking UK   http://www.quitsmokinguk.com
This is a more professional site – an entire portal devoted entirely to those
trying to quit.
Resuscitation Council UK   http://www.resus.org.uk/
SiteIndx.htm

Stroke Association   www.stroke.org.uk
This organisation provides access to information for patients and carers.

Walking the Way to Health Initiative
(WHI)

www.whi.org.uk

Europe

European Heart Journal

http://www.harcourt-international.com/journals/euhj/default.cfm?/

European Heart Network
European Society of Cardiology

http://www.ehnheart.org/
http://www.escardio.org/

USA

Acute Stroke Toolbox
Adult Congenital Heart Association
American Heart Association
American Hypertension Society
Circulation (Journal)
Heart Information Network
HeartPoint
National Heart, Lung and Blood
   Institute
The Heart: an online exploration

www.stroke-site.org
http://www.achaheart.org/
http://www.americanheart.org/
http://www.ash-us.org/
http://circ.ahajournals.org/
http://www.heartinfo.org/
http://www.heartpoint.com/
http://www.nhlbi.nih.gov/index.htm

http://sln.fi.edu/biosci/heart.html

Worldwide

Coronary Health Care (Journal)

http://www.harcourt-international.com/journals/chec/default.cfm

Global Cardiology Network
International Society for Heart
   Research
World Heart Day
World Heart Federation
World Hypertension League

http://www.globalcardiology.org/
http://www.ishrworld.org/

http://www.worldheartday.com/
http://www.worldheart.org/
http://www.mco.edu/whl/

Training programmes

The **British Heart Foundation** runs a programme of training in the secondary prevention of coronary heart disease for nurses working in the community. It is accredited by Buckinghamshire Chilterns University College for 30 CATS points at Level 2.

Apply to the BHF Heart Save Project, University of Oxford, Institute of Health Sciences, Old Road, Headington, Oxford OX3 7LF. Tel: 01865 226975. Fax: 01865 226739. Email: heartsave@dphpc.ox.ac.uk

The **Scottish Heart and Arterial Risk Prevention (SHARP)** course for nurses, includes cardiovascular risk identification, stratification and management. Contact the SHARP Office, University Department of Medicine, Ninewells Hospital and Medical School, Dundee DD1 9SY. Tel: 01382 660111 ext. 33124.

The **British Hypertension Society** Information Service gives advice about local courses on hypertension and CHD risk factors. Tel: 0208 725 3412. Fax: 0208 725 2959.

Index